A CLEAR, CONCISE GUIDE FOR THE PREVENTION AND CONTROL OF HEART DISEASE— AMERICA'S NUMBER ONE KILLER!

- *HOW TO PREVENT HEART ATTACKS*

- *WHAT TO DO AFTER A HEART ATTACK*

- *THE EFFECTS OF DRUGS AND ALCOHOL*

- *SPECIAL EXERCISES AND DIETS*

- *HOW TO BUILD UP YOUR HEART'S RESERVE POWERS*

ADD YEARS TO YOUR HEART

CONTAINS EVERYTHING YOU NEED TO KNOW FOR INCREASING THE LIFE OF THE MOST VITAL ORGAN IN YOUR BODY!

ADD YEARS TO YOUR HEART

A Guide to the Prevention and Control of Heart Disease

DR. MAX WARMBRAND

Author of *The Encyclopedia of Natural Health*

With an Introduction by
HARRY SACKREN, M.D.

PYRAMID BOOKS • NEW YORK

ADD YEARS TO YOUR HEART

A PYRAMID BOOK
Published by arrangement with the author

Pyramid edition published July, 1969
    Second printing April, 1970
    Third printing April, 1971
    Fourth printing September, 1971

Printed in the United States of America

PYRAMID BOOKS are published by Pyramid
Communications, Inc. Its trademark, consisting of the word
"Pyramid" and the portrayal of a pyramid, are registered
in the United States Patent Office.

Pyramid Communications, Inc., 919 Third Avenue,
New York, N.Y. 10022

PREFACE

Time and time again we discover that convictions and beliefs which guide our thinking and action are fallacious.

Albert Schweitzer in his *Out of My Life and Thought* gave us an explanation of why our thinking and action is often motivated in the wrong direction.

"The man of to-day is exposed to influences which are bent on robbing him of all confidence in his own thinking . . . Over and over again convictions are forced upon him in the same way as by means of the electric advertisements which flare in the streets of every large town. Any company which has sufficient capital to get itself securely established, exercises pressure on him at every step he takes to induce him to buy their boot polish or their soup tablets."

It seems to us that many reasons could be advanced for the existence of these misconceptions and that the blame can not be placed solely on one factor.

However, irrespective of the reasons, it should be apparent that only when we can free ourselves completely from the influence of these misconceptions, can we examine each idea on its own merits, and arrive at the truth of any phenomenon.

An investigation of many of our concepts in the realm of health will reveal that here, too, many of the beliefs entertained by vast masses of people are contrary to reason or fact. One of the concepts almost universally accepted, which upon examination is found to be fallacious, is the almost blind belief that medicine provides the answer to disease and suffering.

For thousands of years we have clung to the idea that medicines heal the sick. The sick have multiplied and so have the medicines, which at first the medicineman of

5

ancient times, and more recently the profession of medicine, have been offering us in an ever increasing stream.

Medicines come and go. Each time a new medicine is ushered into the world, it is heralded as the final answer to the sufferings of a large segment of our population. But disillusionment follows disillusionment, and the number of sick keeps increasing from year to year.

As a result of these failures, new concepts are constantly arising, challenging many of the outmoded ideas of the past and rolling up significant successes.

There are nuggets of gold hidden everywhere, but to be able to find them we must be willing to search, keeping our minds free from preconceived notions and beliefs, and be ready to accept values wherever they exist. Such an open-minded and dispassionate approach applied to the problems of health and disease will amply reward us.

CONTENTS

the United States from Coronary Thrombosis. Do Heart Attacks Occur Suddenly? How Children's Lives Have Been Saved. Cholesterol, Cause or Effect? Cholesterol Accumulation, the Result of Impaired Metabolism. Hormone Therapy. Insulin and Diabetes. Cortisone and ACTH. Low Blood Pressure.

The Role of Nutrition in Heart Disease. Why Fat Foods Should Be Excluded. Why Table Salt Is Excluded. How Much Protein Should Be Used. Experiences in Denmark, Great Britain and the United States During World Wars I and II. The Value of the Non-meat Regimen. The Classical Rice Diet. Integrated Nutritional Program Essential. The Superiority of Uncooked Foods. Statement on Nutrition of New York County Medical Society. Deficiencies and Overeating Factors in the Cause of Degenerative Diseases. Rockefeller Foundation Experiments. Importance of Small Meals. Proper Food Preparations. Normal Bowel Functioning. Benefits Derived from Omission of Food.

Report of the Delaney Congressional Committee. The Story of "Agene." Our Experience with Lithium Chloride. The Bread Softeners and Other Chemicals Used in Bread and Cakes Baked Commercially. The Arsenical Sprays. DDT and Virus X. The Harmful Effects of Chlordane. The Benefits Derived from Organically Grown Foods. Hydrochloric Acid Solution to Wash Off Chemicals. Law Regarding Use of Pesticides.

Smoking and Cancer of the Lungs. The Effect of Smoking on the Heart and Circulation. Smoking and the Increase in Mortality. Why Do Doctors Condone Smoking? Our Financial Stake in the Tobacco Industry. Smoking Not the Only Harmful Factor. How to Stop Smoking.

The Effect of Alcohol on the Liver, Digestion and Nerves. The Use of Alcohol in Angina Pectoris. How Alcohol Affects Us When Taken in Small Doses. Tobacco and Alcohol Complementary. The Social Aspects of Tobacco and Alcohol.

INTRODUCTION

In making this timely and well-authenticated plea to the public for a re-evaluation of our approach to the diseases of the heart and the circulatory system, the author of this book is rendering a distinct public service.

Not only has he done an outstanding job of explaining in clear and concise form how these diseases develop; he has also presented a mass of solid and helpful information at a time when it is most needed.

Our approach to the treatment of the sick is in a constant state of flux and changes with the prevailing concepts of the day. Both in theory and practice these changes continue, and what is considered sound practice at one time is often completely discarded at a later period.

However, irrespective of the practices that are being followed at any particular time, the point that must always be kept in mind is that to aid the body in its recovery, the inherent recuperative powers of the patient must be permitted to function freely and unhampered.

The evolution of the school of homeopathy to some degree proved the validity of this approach. Hahneman's superior therapeutic results as compared to those of his contemporaries in the 18th century were attained because his inert medications were not powerful enough to interfere with the patient's recuperative powers and thus did not interfere with recovery.

By the end of the 18th century and during the early part of the 19th century, successful therapy was based largely on the application of Nature's physical forces, such as heat, electricity, muscular activities, hydrotherapy, massage, rest, climate, spa, diet, and general hygienic measures.

This type of therapy arising in reaction to the practice then prevailing which embodied the excessive use of drugs, also proved how superior our results could be when we do not obstruct or retard the body's recuperative functions.

From the end of the 19th century up to our time, medical research concentrated its attention on the specific causes of disease, and encouraged by its success in isolating bacterial agents as the apparent causative factors, broadened its vast fount of knowledge in the sciences of immunology, chemotherapy, anti-biotics, hormones, corticoids, vitamins, etc., in the hope that this would help unlock the door to many of our baffling diseases. Thus, working in this direction, our attention was diverted from the simpler procedures of therapy, and this gave rise to a vast armamentarium of drugs which in most instances are interfering with the innate curative powers of the body and actually are defeating our purpose.

Dealing with the subject of health from a general point of view, we find that while the advance of civilization and the growth of science and technology have brought forth infinite life-enriching values, they have also given rise to practices which have proven highly detrimental to health. The devitaminizing and devitalizing of many of our foods to suit commercial interests and conveniences, the widespread use of the poisonous insecticides in agriculture, the continuous and progressive depletion of our soil, are some of the practices of today which exhaust the nutritional potentialities of our land and ravage our bodies.

The pollution of the air we breathe, the overindulgences which come easy with greater security and comfort, and the hectic life with its noise and bustle are some of the other factors which ruthlessly shorten our lives.

The obligation of the physician to those who seek his advice and guidance should be above all to emphasize the need of avoiding as far as possible all the influences which have a deleterious effect upon the body, and to stress an optimum nutritional program, plus such modifications and adjustments in our habits of living which will raise bodily resistance and fortify us against the impact of unavoidable tensions.

This is the basic thought which has motivated the author in his work and which has earned for him an enviable reputation.

It is now becoming clearly apparent that the trend in the healing professions is rapidly veering in this direction and more and more physicians are now incorporating this approach in their practice.

We can find no quarrel with the author when he emphasizes that diseases of the heart and blood vessels do not develop suddenly but arise gradually as a result of influences which lead to a premature wearing out of the organism and a breakdown of function. His thesis that the elimination of health-destroying habits and the substitution of a sensible way of living offer the best protection against these baffling diseases, permits of no serious contradiction. That these changes can be of material help in the correction of these diseases, is also becoming ever more evident.

With this book, the author has made an important contribution to the literature of health. We physicians would do well to pause and reflect on the author's final statement that only by following such a program can we obtain "the most of health and the best of life."

HARRY SACKREN, M.D.

ACKNOWLEDGMENT

We wish to express our deep appreciation to Jacob M. Leavitt, M.D., Fellow of the American College of Gastroenterology, who despite a very busy practice, has given unstintingly of his time and effort to review all the phases covered in this book and to check its contents for scientific accuracy. Dr. Leavitt's suggestions have been of tremendous help.

We are also deeply grateful to Harry Sackren, M.D., M.P.H., who has devoted a great deal of research in the field of hygienic practice and has cooperated with us for many years in our work.

We are grateful to Dr. Stanley C. Weinsier, resident director of the Florida Spa, closely associated with us for more than forty years, for his help in the assembling of our material, and wish to express our gratitude to Mr. Samuel Rosenbloom and Mr. David Holiday for the splendid job they have done in the editing and correcting of the manuscript.

Furthermore, to all scientists and research workers who are working unceasingly to effect a change in our approach to the diseases of the heart and circulatory system, we express our gratitude.

MAX WARMBRAND, N.D., D.O., D.C.

ADD YEARS TO YOUR HEART

CHAPTER I

OUR GREATEST HEALTH HAZARD

The increase in heart and blood vessel diseases presents us with a challenge of major proportions; a challenge which must be met if millions of lives are to be saved from premature extinction. To highlight the seriousness of the situation, it should be sufficient to mention that well over ten million people in the United States suffer from these diseases and that in 1952, 817,000 died from them— an all time high.

One of the great tragedies in connection with this situation is the fact that so many of those who suffer or die from these diseases are those in the younger age groups or in the very prime of life.

What is even more tragic is the fact that the number of sufferers from these diseases, and the fatalities resulting from them, have been mounting from year to year and are now at their peak, with no hope for relief in sight.

That the situation is critical is well known. *The New York Times* in an editorial (January 13, 1948) pointed out how serious the situation has become when it mentioned that while at the beginning of the century, the mortality from the diseases of the heart and arteries in the City of New York amounted to 118.1 persons per 100,000 population, the number has risen steadily to the point where by 1947 it reached the figure of 400.2 per hundred thousand population.

In other words, the mortality from the diseases of the heart and arteries in the City of New York in the last half century has multiplied almost fourfold.

Dealing with the problem from another aspect, the Mutual Life Insurance Company, in a report based upon a study of one million policy holders, mentioned that we have reached the point where 57 percent of all deaths in all age groups result from diseases of the heart and blood vessels.

Scientists have long been aware of the seriousness of this problem and have been baffled by it. In the 1920's Dr. Haven Emerson, former Commissioner of Health of the City of New York, voiced his concern about the situation and wondered what could be done about it.

Only a few years later Dr. Donald H. Armstrong, Vice President of the Metropolitan Life Insurance Company, referred to the enormity of the problem when he pointed out that the mortality from these diseases in the United States has risen from 111.2 per hundred thousand population in 1900 to 184 per hundred thousand population in 1933.[1]

It was also about the same time that Dr. Jonathan C. Meakins, of Montreal, Canada, President of the College of Physicians, mentioned that "33 percent of deaths of all ages and about one half of deaths at the age of 45 or beyond" were due to the disease of the heart and blood vessels.[2]

The problem has been growing more formidable with each year and has reached a state where, unless a solution is found, it is bound to assume the nature of a major catastrophe.

That most of our health authorities are at a loss and unable to tell how the inroads of these diseases may be checked or be brought under control, is apparent. "We are only at the beginning of advances in knowledge in the field of cardiovascular diseases," stated Dr. Robert L. Levy, President of the New York Heart Association, only a few years ago,[3] while Dr. Alfred E. Cohen, after discussing some of the theories which have been advanced to explain the reason for the rise in these diseases, concluded "that pitifully little is known."[4] Dr. Irving H. Page, one of our leading heart specialists and President of the American Heart Association, pointed out only recently how far we were from a solution of the problem when he

[1] *American Medicine,* 1933.
[2] *New York Times,* April 20, 1934.
[3] *New York Times,* February 15, 1949.
[4] *New York Times,* February 13, 1949.

stated that "Medicine is still getting nowhere in its attack on heart and artery diseases (which cause more than half of all U. S. deaths),"[5] and also mentioned that "when it comes to arteriosclerosis knowledge lags fifty years behind the medical times."[6]

Dr. Paul Dudley White, noted Boston heart specialist, was the latest to acknowledge that we are losing ground in our fight against heart disease, and, furthermore, pointed out "that coronary thrombosis in the United States almost amounted to an 'epidemic'."[7]

However, while the picture at this moment seems admittedly grim, there is no reason for despair since more and more authorities are finally awakening to the realization that only by acquiring a clearer understanding of the underlying causes of these diseases can we come close to a solution of the problem.

When the *New York Times*[8] in a recent editorial mentioned that "there is no certain information on the relation of occupation, stress and strain, diet, habits, the use of alcohol and tobacco to coronary thrombosis" and referred to the statement of Dr. Paul Dudley White that "nobody as yet has made an adequate study of these various underlying factors," it shows that our authorities are now finally beginning to realize the direction in which research has to be channeled if these diseases are to be brought under control.

While this involves a radical departure from the conventional approach, it should be of interest to learn that many authorities are now recognizing the fact that only by a change in our habits of living can the solution to this problem be found.

Dr. Edward L. Bortz,[9] Philadelphia's leading heart specialist and past President of the American Medical Association, has been stressing the importance of these factors for a long time. He mentioned sometime ago that the average person "eats too much of the wrong foods and generally overstuffs, passes up exercise and doesn't bother

[5] *Time,* April 19, 1954.
[6] *New York Times* Editorial, October 2, 1955.
[7] *New York Times,* February 14, 1956.
[8] *New York Times,* October 2, 1955.
[9] *Sunday Compass,* December 4, 1949.

to relax" and that as a result wears out his body thirty years too soon.

He continued further by stating that by correct living man "could live to be 100 easily."

That a change in our mode of living could save many lives and prolong the lives of others by many years is now being recognized to an ever greater extent. When Dr. A. A. Bogomoletz,[10] of recent longevity serum fame, stated that "a man of sixty or seventy is still young, he has lived only half of his natural life," it was not mere conjecture on his part. His statement conformed to the observations of many scientists who, in search of a guide to what our life span could be, noted that animals in their natural state attain a life span of from five to seven times it takes to reach maturity.

Since man reaches maturity at the age of twenty to twenty-five years, it seemed obvious that if we lived in accordance with the laws of nature, our life span, too, could be extended to five to seven times our age at maturity, thus giving us a life span of from 100 to 150 years.

While Dr. Bogomoletz' serum failed to live up to its original promise and has long been forgotten (Bogomoletz himself died at the age of 65 from hardening of the arteries), the idea that our present day life span of 50-80 is not Nature's limit, and can be considerably prolonged, should act as a challenge to all of us.

That we are far from this goal is only too well known. While we continue to boast of the progress we are making, we know that a great many of our people do not even reach the proverbial "three score and ten," but die in the early forties, fifties, or sixties. What is even more tragic is that many of those who die prematurely, suffer for many years from one or more of the many serious metabolic or degenerative diseases which play havoc with our lives. Heart diseases and high blood pressure, cancer, diabetes, the various degenerative diseases of the nervous system, the diseases of the kidneys and the liver, are found rampant, causing untold suffering and shortening the lives of millions of people.

While some of our readers may be skeptical as to

---

[10] *The Prolongation of Life.*

whether our life span could really be extended to between 100 to 150 years, we are certain that most of us would be interested if, by making a few simple readjustments in our habits of living, premature breakdown could be avoided and life could be prolonged.

It is unfortunate that the beginnings of diseases, in most instances, are not easily recognized, and that we become aware that we are ill only when pain or other symptoms of discomfort set in. It is for this reason that the clear relationship between our habits of living and the diseased condition which ultimately makes its appearance is often overlooked. We fail to realize that these diseases are the outgrowth of abuses extending over a period of time, and that only when the abuses which have given rise to them are eliminated can these diseases be checked or modified.

The precious gift of life, free from disease and pain, is within our reach, but can only be attained when we learn to follow a sound program of living.

CHAPTER II

THE FASCINATING STORY
OF THE BLOOD

One of the most fascinating stories of the body is the story of the blood and its circulation. The role of the bloodstream, its composition and its functioning, have interested scientists for many ages. While the bloodstream is the medium through which oxygen and nutrition are carried to the cells and through which their waste products are eliminated, it performs many other valuable functions. It helps to regulate the heat of the body, distribute the secretions of the internal glands, maintain the acid-base balance of the system, and protect the body against what is commonly known as "infection."

That the blood plays an important role in maintaining the health of the body was known long before Dr. Harvey's monumental discovery of the circulation of the blood. However this discovery opened new vistas, helped to clear up many problems and made possible a great deal of additional progress.

Today the importance of the blood and its effect upon our health and well-being are fully recognized, and it is now well known that any impairment in its composition or functioning will vitally affect the body as a whole.

The Composition of the Blood

When we talk of the blood, we talk of a vast world teeming with countless microscopic entities known as the blood cells. This enormous population, confined within the blood vessels, lives and functions in a sea of fluid, known as the plasma. About half our blood is composed of plasma, while the other half is made up of the blood cells which live and work in it.

Two types of blood cells inhabit this strange world—the red and the white. The red blood cells pick up the oxygen in the lungs and carry it to all the cells of the body, while one of the most important functions of the white blood cells is to fight off "infection" or foreign matter.

For one to visualize the prolific life which exists within our bloodstream, it should be sufficient to mention that each cubic millimeter of blood in the average healthy human body contains about five million red blood cells and between 7,500 to 10,000 white blood cells. The count of the red blood cells may vary somewhat with the individual. In women we may find about four and a half million, while in a new-born infant the count may run as high as six to eight million per cubic millimeter.

The count of the white blood cells increases considerably during so-called "infection" and reduces again to normal when the infectious process clears up.

Since the average adult body contains about six to eight quarts of blood, we can readily vizualize that the red and white blood cells, which live and work within the confines of our body, reach astronomical figures.

As is well known, the blood vessels are air-tight to prevent the air from coming in contact with the blood. In case of injury, the blood of a healthy person clots quickly when coming in contact with the air and this seals the wound. The blood contains such clotting substances as thrombin, prothrombin, thromboplasbin, ionized calcium and fibrinogen, which make it clot whenever it comes in contact with air. In case of injury this protects us against hemorrhage.

When some of these elements are not present in the blood in adequate amounts, or when an imbalance exists, the blood may not be able to clot properly, and in case of injury we would be in danger of bleeding to death. On the other hand, under certain conditions the blood may tend to clot too quickly, and we would then be in danger of forming blood clots. This is the condition which exists when clots form in the heart, the brain, or the extremities.

In the healthy body the clotting mechanism is in perfect balance, and the problem of too rapid or incomplete clotting of the blood arises only when our health has become impaired sufficiently to upset this balance.

CHAPTER III

THE HEART—A LIVING PUMP

That the heart and the circulation of the blood play a most vital part in maintaining the health of our body is well known. The living body is a composite of billions of living cells, each cell a microscopic unit of life, each in need of oxygen and food and of disposing its waste products. The cells receive their food and oxygen and eliminate their waste products by way of the blood which is kept in constant circulation by the pumping heart.

The heart is a hollow muscular organ, about the size of a fist. The inner part of the heart is divided into four chambers, two on the right and two on the left side. The upper chambers are separated from the lower chambers by a partition which contains a valve which opens downward. These valves open when the heart muscle relaxes and close when contraction sets in, thus regulating the flow of blood to the body and to the lungs. This process continues without a stop throughout life.

Each side of the heart is completely separate from the other and handles its own particular part of the circulation. As such, the heart may be regarded as a dual pump, taking care of two separate but inter-related circulations.

The right side of the heart pumps the poison-laden and oxygen-deficient blood which is brought back from all over the body, into the lungs, where carbon dioxide is given off and new oxygen is taken on. The left side of the heart receives the purified and oxygen-enriched blood from the lungs and then pumps it into the general circulation for distribution to all parts of the body.

Have you ever watched a pump at work, its piston moving up and down, up and down, at regular, rhythmic intervals? The heart has no piston but, like the pumping engine, keeps pumping steadily, contracting and relaxing its muscular tissue at regular, rhythmic intervals, forcing the flow of blood onward and forward.

Here is a step by step description of how the heart performs its work.

When the poison-laden and oxygen-depleted blood is brought back to the heart, it is first emptied into the upper right chamber. From there it is pumped into the lower right chamber, and then carried by two blood vessels (the pulmonic arteries) into the lungs.

After giving up its carbon dioxide and taking on a new supply of oxygen, it is then carried through an entirely different set of blood vessels—this time four in number, two from each lung—into the left upper chamber of the heart. From there it is pumped into the lower left chamber and then pumped into the general circulation for distribution to all parts of the body.

We have seen that each side of the heart is completely separated from the other. Occasionally, however, we are confronted with a case where an opening exists between the two sides of the heart. This is a mechanical abnormality of congenital origin and is dangerous to life since it permits the blood to seep through in the wrong direction, causing the blood of the two circulations to intermingle. Surgery is now being used in many of these cases as a corrective measure.[1]

The upper chambers of the heart fill with blood during their moment of relaxation and empty their content into the lower chambers during their moment of contraction, both sides performing their work simultaneously.

This work goes on continuously, each pumping beat of the heart, each lub-dub, taking about nine-tenths of a second or about 72 times per minute. It is less when the body is at rest and more when the heart has more work to do.

However, while the heart maintains its work continuously, it also has its periods of rest. It rests between each

---

[1] Where this type of surgery is necessary, the importance of a carefully planned mode of living must be recognized since in addition to correcting the mechanical abnormality, the heart, as well as the rest of the body, must be strengthened so that the patient can come through the operation successfully and be protected against future breakdowns.

beat, and each interval of rest is about twice as long as the beat itself.

With each contraction, the heart pumps about three ounces of venous or oxygen-depleted blood into the lungs, and an equal amount of arterial or oxygen-enriched blood into the general circulation.

The total volume of blood in our body is about six to eight quarts. Since three ounces of blood pass through the heart with each beat and since each beat of the heart takes about 9/10 of a second, the total volume of blood passes through the heart and completes its cycle throughout the body in about one to one and a half minutes.

It is important to bear in mind that while each side of the heart handles its own specific part of the circulation, both sides work in unison. Both upper chambers of the heart fill with blood during their momentary state of expansion and empty their contents into the lower chambers during their moment of contraction.

The lower chambers of the heart also work in team-like fashion. They fill during their momentary state of expansion, and force the blood onward during their moment of contraction.

From the right lower chamber, the oxygen-depleted blood is forced into the lungs for purification and the taking on of new oxygen, while from the left lower chamber the oxygen-enriched blood is pumped into the general circulation for distribution to all parts of the body.

The rapidity or intensity with which the heart works is determined to a great extent by the demand which is placed upon it. When the heart has less work to do, it is more at ease and usually works at a slower pace. When a greater demand is made, it is forced to work at a faster pace and with greater intensity. When an organ is called upon to do more work, it must be supplied with more oxygen, and the heart must pump more blood to supply it. When we run or exercise, more oxygen is needed and the heart is forced to pump harder. The same is true when we eat. To digest the food, the digestive organs require more oxygen, and the heart is called upon to do more work.

More oxygen is required during illness, and this again increases the work of the heart. The same holds true in excitement, tension, overwork, or any type of emotional stress.

When the heart is in a healthy condition, it possesses a great deal of power and strength, providing not only for the regular demands of the body, but also a great deal of reserve to be able to meet unforeseen or unexpected needs.

Whenever a demand for an increase in circulation arises anywhere in the body, this demand is transmitted with lightning speed to the pumping mechanism of the heart and when the heart is in good health, it unfailingly responds to this need.

It should be apparent, however, that whenever the heart is called upon to spend its reserve powers recklessly, it will ultimately become worn out and its efficiency and power will become impaired.

These reserve powers should be husbanded carefully so that they may be at our disposal during periods of actual stress, as in the case of disease, accident, or shock, and it is the height of folly to squander them carelessly, thereby jeopardizing our health and our life.

That the normal heart possesses amazing functional and recuperative powers is well known. Scientific writers often overwhelm us with their description of the amount of work the heart can do and marvel at the precision with which it performs its functions. However, it is the rare scientist who points out that even this powerful organ can ultimately become weakened and worn out, and that to protect ourselves against this possibility, our reserve powers must not be needlessly drawn upon.

At this point, it is well to mention that since the heart, too, is composed of living tissue, it, also, must receive nutrition and oxygen, if it is to keep well and be able to do its work. However, it is of interest to know that the nutrient elements and oxygen which the heart receives are not obtained by it from the blood which passes through it during its pumping operation, but from the blood which is supplied to it through a special set of arteries—the coronary arteries.

The coronary arteries are the first two arteries which branch off from the main arterial trunk as it emerges from the lower left chamber of the heart, and then divides in many smaller branches carrying blood to all parts of the heart.

CHAPTER IV

THE ARTERIES AND VEINS

While the work of the heart is to pump the blood and keep it in circulation, the work of the arteries is to carry the blood with its oxygen and other nutrient materials to every cell and part of the body.

The arteries are composed of soft, elastic muscle fibres and are powerful enough to take the full impact of the pumping heart in its stride. They expand to receive the blood which the heart pumps into them and contract to force it onward.

Since the arteries are composed of living tissue, they also require food and oxygen, but just as in the case of the heart, they obtain their nutrients not from the blood which flows through them, but from the blood which is brought to them by their own special arteries, the *vaso vasorum*. An intricate system of nerves plays an important part in regulating their function.

Starting with the main artery, the aorta, which emerges from the lower left chamber of the heart, the arterial system branches into a vast network of large and small arteries, reaching out in every direction and carrying blood with its oxygen and other nutrient elements to every cell and part of the body. The large arteries subdivide first into smaller arteries, then into still smaller arteries, and finally into the minute, hairlike blood vessels known as the capillaries.

The Capillaries

We have seen that one of the main functions of the blood is to supply food and oxygen to the cells and to carry off their waste products. However, it is necessary to point out that the actual interchange between the blood and the tissue cells takes place not in the large arteries or their smaller subdivisions, but in their smallest subdivisions, the capillaries. The capillaries are the minute, thin-walled hairlike channels stretching many thousands of miles, reaching into every nook and corner of the body, carrying food and oxygen to all the cells of the body and removing their waste products.

This interchange between the capillaries and the tissue cells takes place through the very thin walls of the capillaries and proceeds at billions of different points simultaneously.

This process of interchange is known as osmosis, and may be compared to the transposition which takes place when two liquids, one containing salt, the other sugar, are separated from one another by a thin, permeable membrane. A reciprocal exchange of the contents of both solutions takes place and the contents of both solutions become equalized. This is how the exchange between the cells and the blood takes place. The cells take the oxygen and other essential elements out of the blood, and in turn give up their waste products.

It is not always easy for the human mind to visualize the minuteness of a capillary. Kahn[1] states that each capillary is "fifty times finer than the finest human hair," and points out that it is so minute that about 700 capillaries could be packed into the space occupied by the thickness of a pin.

In other words, a capillary would have to be magnified 700 times to equal the thickness of a pin.

Through these tiny microscopic blood vessels the blood corpuscles pass steadily in single file, carrying oxygen and other nutritive elements to the cells, and carrying off their toxins.

The capillaries, the smallest subdivision of the arteries, also form the beginning of the veins. Neighboring capillaries merge and form small veins, *venulea,* out of which by fusion the larger veins are formed.

---

[1] Fritz Kahn, *Man in Structure and Function.*

The Veins

While the arteries carry the oxygen-enriched blood to the cells, the veins carry the oxygen-depleted and poison-laden blood back to the right side of the heart to be pumped into the lungs for purification and re-oxygenation. However, even though both types of blood vessels are part of the same circulatory system, they nevertheless show certain structural differences. The arteries, closer to the pumping heart and exposed to its full force, have a much heavier load to carry and because of this are more powerfully developed and possess a greater resiliency than the veins.

The veins, on the other hand, possess a unique feature which is not found in the arteries. They are covered with valves to prevent the blood from flowing back. The veins, being farther away from the heart and not benefitting to the same degree as the arteries from its pumping force or "push," need this added protection.

The Kidneys—Part of a Trinity

The kidneys, too, bear an important relationship to the heart and blood vessels. They are part of a trinity which together control circulation and affect the health of the body. While the heart acts as the pump which maintains the circulation and the arteries provide the channels through which the blood circulates, the kidneys are the organs which filter the toxic wastes from the blood.

Another important function of the kidneys is to control the fluid content of the body. About two-thirds of the human body is composed of fluids. The cells contain fluids and live in a fluid medium. The blood, too, is largely composed of fluids.

We take fluid into our system with our food and drink, and have to eliminate that which the body is unable to use. Some of it is expelled through the lungs in the form of vapor, when we exhale. We excrete quite a bit through our sweat glands, but the greatest portion is usually eliminated through the kidneys.

The kidneys have an elaborate filter system composed of

miles and miles of hair-sized filtering tubules. In one day, many quarts of fluid pass through these filters, but the greatest amount is reabsorbed by the tubules and only about one to two quarts are actually eliminated through the kidneys.

When the kidneys become damaged, they are unable to filter out the wastes from the blood and the intricate mechanism which controls the fluid content of the body is unable to function efficiently. This upsets the equilibrium in the body and places an increased burden on the heart and the blood vessels.

How important the function of the kidneys is to the maintenance of health can be seen from the fact that approximately twenty percent of all the blood pumped by the heart is carried to the kidneys.

When the heart is damaged, the kidneys fail to receive an adequate supply of blood and this in turn impairs the intricate filtering mechanism and upsets the fluid balance. As a result, fluids begin to accumulate in the system, appearing first in the area of poorest circulation, the feet and legs, and then, as the disease progresses, in the abdomen and chest. The retention of this fluid places an added load on an already overworked heart and may ultimately progress to the point where the patient virtually drowns in his own fluids.

It should be apparent from all this that the workings of the heart, the blood vessels and the kidneys are closely inter-related, and that damage to one organ will adversely affect the function of the others.

CHAPTER V

THE THREE MAJOR TYPES
OF HEART DISEASE

The types of heart disease which are most prevalent and which take the greatest toll of human life may be grouped in the following three categories:

1. HYPERTENSIVE HEART DISEASE

Hypertensive heart disease is the type of heart disease which develops as a result of, or in connection with, high blood pressure. When the blood pressure is high, the heart is forced to work harder to maintain the circulation. In order to cope with this added demand, the muscle of the heart is forced to enlarge.

While an enlargement of the heart is a characteristic sign in this type of heart disease, it must be remembered that a mere enlargement in the size of the heart is not in itself an indication of heart disease. Athletes, or physically active persons, often develop larger heart muscles as a result of their physical activities. However, a muscle which becomes larger because of normal physical exertion is a healthy muscle, while a muscle which is forced to enlarge when too much work is thrust upon it is sapped of its strength and ultimately becomes worn out and damaged.

Arteriosclerosis or Hardening of the Arteries

There are many factors which contribute to the development of high blood pressure. Nervous tension, glandular disorders, certain types of kidney disease, and a change in the volume or consistency of the blood, are among them. However, the factor which most often contributes to it is hardening of the arteries.

We have seen that the arteries in the healthy individual are soft and pliable and are able to expand and contract effectively. When the arteries become hard and brittle and the inner walls thicken and narrow, they are unable to do their work efficiently, and the heart is forced to pump much harder to maintain circulation.

Hardening of the arteries occurs in two forms. One, the stempipe or calcifying type of hardening, is caused by the gradual deposit of calcium within the walls of the arteries. While this condition is found most frequently in older people, the young are not immune to it. The other, the cholesterol type of hardening, develops when cholesterol, a chemical substance of fatty origin, deposits within the walls of the arteries.

When cholesterol accumulates in an artery, sores or ulcers develop at the site of deposit, and in time this is followed by hardening and thickening. This change narrows the channel through which the blood flows and ultimately leads to the formation of clots.

Since this type of hardening affects the younger age groups most frequently and takes the greatest toll of life from among the young and those in the prime of life, this is the type of hardening which is of greatest concern to us.

What Is Blood Pressure?

When we talk of blood pressure, we talk of the pressure exerted within the blood vessels by the circulating blood. The blood pressure is measured to determine the amount of effort exerted by the heart to maintain circulation and the amount of pressure that exists in the arteries when the heart is at rest.

When the heart is in action the pressure is known as the "systolic pressure" and is the higher reading of the two. The pressure when the heart is at rest is the "diastolic pressure." While both pressures are important, the diastolic pressure is the more important as an index of normality since it indicates the degree of tension or strain existing in the circulatory system.

Blood pressure is measured by wrapping an air-tight rubber cuff around the arm. The cuff is then inflated with air until the pulse at the wrist is completely obliterated. When this point is reached, the air is slowly released, permitting the flow of blood to return. The first pulse beat felt at the wrist, or the first throbbing sound heard with a stethoscope at the large artery in the crook of the arm, represents the systolic blood pressure.

As the air is gradually released, the sound again is obliterated. At this point we have what is known as the diastolic pressure.

The blood pressure fluctuates in accordance with the influences which affect the body as a whole. The same influences which affect the heart also affect the blood pressure. Nonetheless, it is of interest to know that blood pressure varies considerably in different parts of the body. It is highest in the arteries nearest the heart and diminishes as we get farther away from the heart. It is lower in the veins than in the arteries.

A mere fluctuation or a temporary rise in blood pressure need not cause alarm. It merely means that some tension or weakening influence has disturbed the normal rhythm and brought about a temporary rise or fall. To determine whether a given blood pressure is normal or not, the reading must be evaluated in relation to the other conditions in the body and to the influences which affect the heart and nervous system at the time the blood pressure is taken.

Authorities disagree as to what the normal blood pressure is. Some maintain that a 100 plus age is normal. Others claim that the normal blood pressure is 100 plus age up to 20 years, and then one point for every two years.

Actually neither of these formulae is completely correct, not merely because blood pressure varies with the individual and fluctuates in accordance with the many influences which affect the heart and the nervous system, but also because both of these formulae assume that blood pressure has to increase with age.

This is not true. While blood pressure tends to rise with age, this is not to be regarded as a normal condition. It occurs because as people grow older, their blood vessels tend to lose some of their elasticity. This, however, need not happen since the blood vessels can be kept pliable and resilient maintaining the blood pressure in the "younger age" range, even as we grow older.

Dr. Harvey Kellogg, founder of the famous Battle Creek Sanitarium, has been known to have a blood pressure of 118/80 at the age of 72 and we have known many other people who at a ripe old age have shown a similar youthful type of blood pressure.

Assuming that these people are otherwise in good health, this merely means that they have a young person's blood pressure.

When Clots Form

In the healthy person, the inner lining of the arteries is smooth and flexible and the blood can flow through them easily. But, as seen before, when calcium or the fat-like substance, cholesterol, deposits on the walls of the arteries, the arteries become hard and brittle, and the channel through which the blood flows becomes narrower. This slows down the circulation of the blood and in time may cause the formation of a clot, obstructing the circulation completely.

When this happens in the brain, we develop what is known as apoplexy or a "stroke." The affected part of the brain fails to receive its supply of blood and the part of the body which is controlled by this part of the brain becomes paralyzed. Whether and to what extent the paralysis clears up depends upon how rapidly and how thoroughly the clot can be reabsorbed. Where the clot fails to be reabsorbed quickly, the part of the brain which fails to get its needed oxygen and nourishment becomes damaged, and the paralysis becomes permanent.

When a clot forms in an artery in the leg, it causes severe cramp-like pains and ultimately leads to a dying (necrosis) of the part which is deprived of its circulation. Gangrene often develops and amputation may become necessary.

Coronary Thrombosis

When a clot forms in one of the arteries of the heart, we have a "coronary thrombosis" or "coronary occlusion." In this condition, the affected part of the heart is deprived of its circulation, and failing to get its nourishment and oxygen, ceases to function. This is known as a typical heart attack.

When the circulation to the kidneys becomes affected, their functions become seriously impaired. They are unable to eliminate the toxins effectively, and the fluid balance in the body becomes upset. This in turn overtaxes the arteries and the heart, and leads to their breakdown.

2. CORONARY OR ARTERIOSCLEROTIC HEART DISEASE

While hypertensive heart disease arises from a general hardening of the arteries or high blood pressure, coronary or arteriosclerotic heart disease develops from a hardening of the coronary arteries, the arteries which supply the heart with its blood supply.

We have seen before that all parts of the body must receive oxygen and nourishment and must dispose of their waste products. The heart is no exception to this rule. However, just as in the case of the arteries, the heart does not obtain its oxygen and other essential nutrition elements from the blood which is pumped through it, but through a special set of arteries, the coronary arteries. These arteries are the first two arteries which branch off from the main arterial trunk as it emerges from the heart and are known as the coronary arteries because of their crown-like formation. These two arteries divide into countless smaller branches and spread out into every part of the heart structure.

Coronary Sclerosis

Coronary or arteriosclerotic heart disease begins with hardening of the coronary arteries. When the coronary arteries become hardened, the condition is known as "coronary sclerosis." When this condition develops, the heart is unable to receive an adequate supply of oxygen and other essential nutritious elements and ultimately begins to break down. Since this condition usually develops slowly and insidiously, the early stages are often not easily recognized. However, as the disease progresses, certain warning symptoms or disturbances often begin to show up. Among these are heaviness or pressure on the chest, or severe excruciating pains in which the chest feels as if it were tightly clamped in a vise, squeezing all life and strength from it.

During these attacks, the pains often radiate into the left shoulder, sometimes into the right shoulder, occasionally into the abdomen.

These attacks are known as angina pectoris and occur when one of the coronary arteries is in spasm because of an insufficient supply of oxygen.

It is fortunate that these attacks last only for a short time, usually no longer than a few seconds, sometimes one or two minutes, rarely more than ten or fifteen minutes. Where they continue for more than a half hour, a coronary thrombosis or coronary occlusion must be seriously suspected.

Coronary Artery Thrombosis

In coronary thrombosis complete obstruction of one of the branches of the coronary arteries has set in. This condition develops when a clot forms blocking the circulation to the affected part of the heart.

A coronary thrombosis often sets in with catastrophic suddenness. In addition to the excruciating pains which persist without letup, some of the other symptoms are considerable difficulty in breathing and acute collapse. The face becomes bathed in sweat and turns ashen gray, and the afflicted has a feeling of impending death.

The patient may in the words of Boyd[1] be "well one minute and in agony the next."

A point to bear in mind, however, is that while the

[1] Boyd, *Pathology of Internal Diseases.*

attack may come on with dramatic suddenness, the disease itself does not develop suddenly, but builds up over a long period of time, and is the outgrowth of blood vessel disease which has become continuously more severe.

The excruciating pains in coronary thrombosis are akin to those of a severe angina pectoris attack, with the only difference that while in an angina attack they subside after a short period of time, in coronary thrombosis the pains persist continuously without a letup.

The sharp excruciating pains which occur in coronary thrombosis or during an angina attack, often radiate into the abdomen and may occasionally be mistaken for indigestion, a perforated ulcer, a gall bladder distress, or a diseased pancreas.

"Under those circumstances, unless the possibility of coronary artery occlusion is kept in mind, it is easy to see how the abdomen may be opened with unfortunate consequences," Boyd warns.

While an attack of coronary thrombosis is of a grave nature, it should not be regarded as hopeless. Many sufferers recover from it and many return to a normal life. The seriousness of the case and the degree of recovery, however, depend upon the extent of involvement and the type of care the patient receives.

Where one of the smaller blood vessels is involved, a smaller area of the heart is affected and the danger is not too great. Where a larger blood vessel is affected, the attack is much more serious and may even result in sudden death.

When an artery becomes obstructed, the part of the heart which fails to receive oxygen dies. However, as soon as this happens the body begins to marshal its forces in an attempt to repair the damage. The dead tissue is softened and carried away and the damaged area fills up with scar tissue.

Of extreme interest at this point is the fact that new blood vessels shoot out from adjacent arteries to carry on the work of the damaged artery. This is known as the collateral circulation and plays an important role in repairing the damage.

Our task during this critical period is to provide that care which will enable the body to do an effective job of repair and of rebuilding the strength of the heart. However, even when this has been accomplished the job is not completed. The patient must be made to realize how the condition developed and the adjustments he must make to protect himself against a reoccurrence.

Sufferers from coronary scleroris (hardening of the arteries of the heart) are committing a grave error when they fail to recognize the seriousness of their condition and do not make an effort to make the necessary adjustments in their habits of living. They must realize that by neglecting to do this they fail to check the inroads of the disease and actually expose themselves more readily to a coronary thrombosis. It is amazing to note that even many of those who have already suffered from an attack of coronary thrombosis often disregard these warnings and fail to make the changes which would protect them against a possible reoccurrence.

While the onset of coronary thrombosis is, in most instances, associated with excruciating pain, an attack may occur without suffering, merely attended by difficulty in breathing and then collapse. This happens when the nerves of the heart have become so badly damaged by a previous attack of coronary thrombosis that they are unable to transmit the sensation of pain.

3. VALVULAR OR RHEUMATIC HEART DISEASE

Valvular or rheumatic heart disease is another type of heart disease which takes a terrific toll of human life. In this type of heart disease, the valves of the heart have become thickened and scarred, and are unable to close or open completely. As a result, some of the blood leaks through or is pushed backward. This disrupts the normal circulation and places a great strain upon the heart. To cope with this condition, the heart is forced to enlarge and because of the added strain, it ultimately becomes worn out.

Fortunately, a great deal of repair is possible in many cases. Proper care strengthens the heart and promotes the necessary readjustments which enable it to function better in spite of the damage.

While the damage in valvular or rheumatic heart disease can be readily discerned, the damage in hypertensive or coronary heart disease, especially during the earlier stages, is not always easily recognized. A physical examination will disclose the presence of an enlarged heart, but cannot always indicate how tired out the heart is or whether hardened or scar tissue exists.

Boyd describes this condition as follows: "Apart from this fibrosis (scar tissue) which may be minimal in degree, the heart muscle appears normal. The individual fibres are healthy and show no suggestion of degeneration."

And yet while apparently normal, in reality the heart does not possess its full strength and clearly shows the effects of wear and tear. Boyd aptly explains, "What seems to be a powerful muscle is unable to expel the blood from the heart with any vigor. The pathologist has to accept the fact that in the myocardium (heart muscle) morphological (structural) appearance does not necessarily correspond with functional capacity."

In other words, even though the heart appears normal it is actually unable to maintain an efficient circulation.

It is well to keep this fact in mind because many people assume that once they have had their periodic health checkup and have been told that their heart is in good condition, they have nothing about which to be concerned. Many of us know of people who were examined by heart specialists and were told that their heart was in good condition, yet died from a heart attack soon after.

In more advanced cases, the damage and worn out condition is, of course, more easily recognized since by that time sufficient degenerative changes have already set in to make the damage apparent. Such changes as a wasting or shrinking of the heart muscle, advanced stages of fatty degeneration, or infiltration of fatty deposits in the heart muscle fibres, are more easily recognized, and many abnormal symptoms such as difficult breathing, night asthma, rapid or slow pulse, swelling of the liver, fluid in the abdomen and chest, help one to make a correct diagnosis.

We are not often aware of this, but such mild disturbances as dizziness, blurred vision or digestive distress, often arise from a minor heart damage. In some cases, several such areas of minor damages become confluent and cause a major defect, leading to so-called "sudden" death. While the sudden death in these cases is due to

43

a major organic breakdown, it is really the outgrowth of a slow form of deterioriation which has reached its peak.

Failure Affects Both Sides of the Heart

When doctors discuss a heart case, they often mention left side failure or right side failure, implying that either one or the other side of the heart has broken down and is unable to do its work. In reality, there is no breakdown which limits itself exclusively to one side of the heart. Failure in most cases begins with the left side but, unless quickly relieved, will affect the right side as well. When the left side of the heart is unable to pump the blood it receives from the lungs, the lungs cannot empty any more blood into it, and as a result there is a backing up to the right side of the heart. The engorgement that results causes a stretching or dilating of the heart and causes many of the difficulties which we have described.

Heart Block

One of the conditions often found in the later stages of heart disease is known as a heart block. We have seen that the function of the heart is in perfect balance. This balance or rhythm is maintained by the nervous system and a special control in the heart muscle, the Sinus rhythm. When this special control becomes impaired, an imbalance between the upper and lower chambers of the heart develops. While the upper chambers function at a normal range, the lower chambers are unable to keep in step. This manifests itself in a slowing of the pulse.

However, a slow pulse is not necessarily a sign of a diseased heart. When a normal heart is at rest, its pulse too slows down, and this is an indication that the heart is merely working at a slower rate and is conserving its energy.

CHAPTER VI

METABOLISM—
A FACTOR IN HEART DISEASE

While diseases of the heart and blood vessels have been increasing at an enormous rate, and while the search for the cause of these diseases and the reason for their continuous increase has been going on for a long time, our research workers, so far, have accomplished very little.

However, a profound change has recently taken place, which if carried to its logical conclusion, holds significant promise for the future. This change took place when our scientists began to realize that diseases of the heart and the circulation arise from an impairment in the metabolism of the body.

The term metabolism covers a wide field. It embraces all the known and unknown functions of the body and all the known and unknown chemical and physiological processes which break down our food and oxygen so that they can be utilized by the cells for the liberation of energy and the rebuilding of our tissues.

The living body is a complex mechanism and its many functions such as the digestion and assimilation of food, the secretion of the endocrine glands, the functions of the nervous system, the elimination of toxins, as well as the thousand and one chemical and physiologic changes which take place continuously within our organism, are part of this complexity.

Anything which impairs these functions leads to a derangement in nutrition, affects the elimination of toxins, impairs glandular functions and causes a chemical imbalance. These are the impairments which exist and which are part and parcel of our so-called "metabolic" diseases.

Diabetes, arthritis, diseases of the kidneys and liver, the various degenerative nervous disorders, as well as the diseases of the heart and blood vessels, all belong in this category.

Our Kidneys—A Vast Filtering System

We have mentioned that the function of our kidneys plays a vital role in the development of high blood pressure and heart disease. The type of kidney disease which contributes to the development of these diseases is known as "glomerular nephritis." The glomeruli are the filters of the kidneys. Each kidney contains billions of these tiny, microscopic filters whose job it is to filter out the fluids and expel the waste products from the body.

It is interesting to mention that while this immense filtering system filters out as much as 185 quarts of fluid from the blood in a single day, about 183½ quarts are reabsorbed into the blood and only about 1½ quarts are eliminated in the form of urine. The amount may vary with the intake of fluid, and varies in certain diseases.

When the kidneys become impaired, they are unable to function efficiently, and as a result, many of the toxins are retained in the system and the fluid balance in the body becomes disrupted. This places an added strain on the heart and raises the blood pressure.

The kidneys break down from overwork or when they have to rid the body of an excessive amount of noxious or irritating substances which have been taken into the system with food or drink, or in the form of drugs or chemicals.

The kidneys are not the only organs which become impaired in this way. The liver, the heart, the blood vessels, the digestive system, in fact any organ or set of organs, can become damaged in the same way and from the same influences.

In his discussion of the diseases of the liver, Boyd[1] expressed this point most vividly when, in explaining how the diseases of the liver arise, he stated:

"The cells of the liver are bathed in the blood brought by the portal vein from the gastro-intestinal tract, blood

[1] Boyd, *Pathology of Internal Diseases.*

which may contain toxins known and unknown. The result of such toxic action may be the death of some or many of the cells of the liver lobule, it may be one or many of the lobules themselves." Then he continues:

"Among the numerous agents most diverse in character, which may cause degeneration and necrosis of liver cells may be mentioned chemicals, both organic and inorganic, certain drugs and tar-like substances (coal tar products), foreign proteins and products of protein decomposition, bacterial toxins, infections, and exposure to radiation."

A moment's thought should make us realize that this explanation could apply with equal emphasis to the diseases of the kidneys, the heart, the arteries, or, for that matter, of any organ or part of the body.

Damage to any organ or tissues of the body results from overwork or is caused by toxins which are generated within the body or find their way into the system from without, with our food or drink or in the form of drugs or chemicals.

It is highly gratifying to note that this concept is now gaining rapid recognition in medical thinking. The credit for this belongs to Dr. Hans Selye, Director of the Institute of Experimental Medicine and Surgery at the University of Montreal, the originator of the theory of "Stress." Dr. Selye has clearly demonstrated that stress and strain, or, in other words, excessive wear and tear, caused by overwork or the accumulation of toxins or substances of an irritating nature which are generated within the system as a result of improper functioning, or which are taken into the system with improper food and drink or in the form of drugs or chemicals, cause disorders in metabolism which ultimately manifest themselves in one or other of our metabolic diseases, the diseases of the heart and blood vessels included.

In other words, anything which overtaxes the organism impairs it functioning and brings about the onset of these diseases.

Health, An Orderly Harmonious Functioning

Health is an orderly, harmonious functioning of all the organs of the body, and this state of harmony continues as long as they are able to do their work efficiently. As an added protection against a disruption of this harmony, our body possesses a tremendous amount of reserve power which is drawn upon in case of stress or difficulties. It is only when these reserve powers have become greatly depleted that the organs are unable to function efficiently and finally break down.

Selye demonstrated this most conclusively. He has shown that whenever our body is subjected to stress of any sort, an alarm reaction immediately arouses the body's reserve powers, calling upon them to cope with the existing strain and restore balance.

However, when the disruptive influences continue unabated or reoccur at frequent intervals, the reserve powers ultimately become exhausted, depleting the margin of safety which protects the body against deterioration and breakdown.

That the body possesses the power to maintain normal harmonious functioning even under stress is not a new idea. Selye refers us to the work of the French physiologist, Claude Bernard, who called attention to the fact that the body maintains its own internal balance. Our own Walter Cannon called this the "homeostasis" (stability or equilibrium) of the body.

Commenting on the work of these well known investigators, Selye pointed out that our life becomes endangered when its reserve powers have become depleted and its ability to make these life-saving adjustments or adaptations has been destroyed or lost.

Selye has merely confirmed what other investigators have long ago suspected, namely, that the glands of internal secretion and the nervous system act as the balance wheels which maintain this equilibrium and protect us against collapse. He has demonstrated that when our body is exposed to stress, it arouses an increase in the secretions of our glands which counteracts the effect of stress and protects us against breakdown.

However, when stress continues over a long period of time, or in excess of what our body can safely handle, the ability of the glands to pour out these life-saving secretions becomes impaired and the body is unable to make the necessary adjustments. When this happens, our health and life are endangered.

Changes in Heart Disease—
Part of This Adaptive Mechanism

It is interesting to note that the changes which take place in heart disease also develop when the body attempts to cope with conditions or influences which threaten life and as such are part of our defense mechanism. We have seen that when the heart has more work to do than it can safely handle, its muscle is forced to enlarge, and that this change takes place to enable the heart to cope with the increased amount of work and to protect it against collapse.

When the blood vessels become thickened and hardened, or when scar tissue develops in the muscle or in and around the valves of the heart, these changes too arise from an attempt to repair an inflamed or damaged area, and to limit the damage from spreading.

The ability of the body to make these repairs, even though they bring with them an alteration in structure, is instrumental in saving human life.

Can Hardening of the Arteries Be Avoided?

While most authorities are profoundly concerned with the increase in the diseases of the heart and the arteries, some try to minimize the seriousness of the situation by telling us that since most people live longer now than ever before, an increase in the incidence and mortality from these diseases is to be expected.

Dr. Walter Modell is one of those who stressed this view only a few years ago. "We have more heart disease today because our health is improving. It is paradoxical that we should seek to find comfort in the statement that more people than ever are dying of heart disease, but it is nevertheless a comforting fact to the physician. He knows that because of the dramatic reduction in deaths caused by infectious diseases, people are in general living much longer. Hardening of the arteries or arterio-sclerosis, the most frequent cause of heart disease, comes to more people today because it eventually comes to all who live long enough."[2]

[2] Dr. Walter Modell, "Straight Facts About Heart Disease," *Hygeia,* Feb. 1948.

At first glance this reasoning may sound plausible. Further examination, however, discloses how fallacious it is. Two major flaws exist in this type of thinking. One is the assumption that people in general live much longer than before. This is not true even though most people have come to believe it.

The other is the assumption that "hardening of the arteries eventually comes to all who live long enough" and is, therefore, inevitable.

An examination of the facts will reveal that neither of these assumptions is true. The life span of our adult population, in spite of all propaganda to the contrary, has really not been considerably prolonged, while hardening of the arteries is not "inevitable" in the older population.

There is no question that the over-all life span of our population has been considerably extended in the last half century, but this does not mean that our adult population is living much longer than fifty years ago. We are not ungrateful even for little favors, but we really have not much to be grateful for insofar as this claim is concerned. An examination of the facts will reveal that the increase we boast of resulted primarily from a saving of infants' and children's lives, and not at all or only to a very limited degree from the prolongation of the life span of our adult population.

The weekly *U. S. News & World Report*[3] in dealing with this question proved this quite clearly. Quoting the U. S. Public Health Service, this weekly disclosed that while the over-all life span in the last half century of an average boy at birth has increased by eighteen years, the life span of a man aged forty, has increased by not more than three years.

The claim that our life span has been extensively prolonged has been repeated at various times but many of our authorities have pointed out how baseless this claim is.

Dr. I. Dublin,[4] Chief Statistician of the Metropolitan Life Insurance Company, referred to this as early as 1928 when, in an address before the New York Academy of Medicine, he pointed out that while more people are living

---

[3] *U. S. News & World Report,* March 24, 1950.
[4] *New York Times,* October 2, 1928.

to an old age, "this has simply been due to the fact that we are saving more lives at younger ages . . .

"A man has practically no more expectation of living beyond 70 now than he had in 1840," he stressed.

Somewhat later we find Alexis Carrel dealing with the same subject. In his book, *Man the Unknown,* published in 1935, he stated, "In spite of the progress achieved in heating, ventilation and lighting of homes, of dietary hygiene, bathrooms and sports, of periodical medical examinations and increasing number of specialists, not even one day has been added to the span of life."

That the increase in the life span of the adult population is more apparent that real can be seen when we examine the facts presented in one of the more recent bulletins published by the Metropolitan Life Insurance Company. In its bulletin, "A Century of Progress in Longevity" (Vol. 50, October 1949), the Metropolitan Life Insurance Company disclosed that while the over-all life expectancy at birth has increased from 49 to 68 years, the life span of a man aged 40 has increased to less than three years and the life span of a man aged 50, barely to two years.

The Brookings Institution[5] also confirmed this point. In an analysis issued recently, the institution disclosed that while the average death rate in the United States in the past 50 years has been reduced from 17.2 per thousand persons in 1900 to 9.6 per thousand persons in 1950, the greatest reduction has taken place in our infant and child population.

Elaborating further on their findings, the Brookings Institution pointed out that the death rate of infants under one year of age in 1900 was 162.4 per thousand live births, and that this has been reduced to 31.3 per thousand live births, or practically 1/5 of what it was at the turn of the century. Continuing further, they mentioned that while the life expectancy at the age of 50 has risen from 59 percent in 1901 to 80 percent in 1950, this resulted primarily from a reduction in the mortality of infants and children, as well as our younger generation, and only to an extremely limited degree, because of an improvement in life expectancy of the adult population.

[5] *New York Times,* August 11, 1952.

Hardening of the Arteries Not Inevitable

That hardening of the arteries is an inevitable process of aging and unavoidable has been repudiated by some of our most noted authorities.

Dealing with this subject, Dr. Joseph D. Wassersug stated: "It would be a mistake to believe that hardening of the arteries is simply part of the general process of aging, and to accept it as such with resignation. On the contrary, scientists are quick to point out that many octogenarians and non-octogenarians die with a minimal amount of sclerosis in their blood vessels whereas fatal amounts are not infrequently noted in early youth and even childhood. To regard hardening of the arteries as a phenomenon inevitably associated with the process of growing old would be deplorable."

Dr. Irving H. Page[6] stated: "Hypertension is certainly not merely a problem of aging. Nor is it a disease exclusively of the aged. It is not sufficiently realized by the public that it is sometimes found even in babies, and that young people in the twenties often have it. It increases in frequency from 30 years on, and is very common in the age period of greatest productivity and usefulness to society."

A recent statement refuting this assertion most emphatically was issued by Doctors Howard B. Burchell, Edgar V. Allen, and Frederick P. Moersch. In an article appearing in the *Journal of the American Medical Association*, these eminent physicians declared that they too desire "to join in the crusade against the teaching of a close relationship between age and arterio-sclerosis, which is either accepted or implied in past medical school curriculums," and then significantly concluded:

"For the purposes of emphasis, let us make the provocative statement that while aging is relentless, arterio-sclerosis is not necessarily a progressive nor irreversible process."[7]

[6] *Hypertension, A Manual for Patients with High Blood Pressure.*

[7] "Clinical Manifestations of Arterio-Sclerosis," Dec. 15, 1951.

Dr. Shirley M. Wynne, Commissioner of Health of the City of New York, long ago recognized the fallacy of this reasoning. While accepting the fact that because more children grow up to adulthood, an increase in the number of degenerative diseases was to be expected, he nevertheless stated:

"This fact, however, cannot entirely account for the situation. The degenerative diseases are increasing at a more rapid rate than is the older population. That is to say, among 1000 older persons, cancer and diabetes, for example, are more prevalent today than they were among 1000 such persons forty to fifty years ago."[8]

What challenges this reasoning to an even greater degree is the fact that the number of heart and circulatory diseases has increased to a greater extent not in the older population but in the younger age groups or those in the prime of life.

Dr. Paul Dudley White[9] in the *Journal of the American Medical Association,* June 28, 1952, in discussing the progress made in the treatment of these diseases stated:

"Despite all these advances, the incidence and mortality rates of cardio-vascular-renal diseases have increased enormously, far more than those of cancer. . . . Of all deaths in the United States, 51 percent can be attributed to cardio-vascular-renal diseases" and then goes on to say that "the situation would not be so discouraging" if only our old persons died from these diseases.

"Unfortunately, however, at present the increase in mortality from cardio-vascular disease does not occur only in old persons. There has been a great increase of the disease in young adults and those of middle age within the last half generation. There is actually a greater increase in these middle years between 30 and 60 than in the later ages."

When Dr. White was called to attend President Eisenhower during his recent heart attack, he pointed out that these attacks are quite common by the time we reach fifty, but rightfully stated that they do not occur suddenly, but are the outgrowth of degenerative changes in the arteries going on over many years.

---

[8] *New York World,* May 25, 1930.
[9] "Heart Disease Forty Years Ago and Now."

Dr. E. Cowle Andrus[10] of Johns Hopkins University, President of the American Heart Association, looking at the situation optimistically, stated that "65 to 70 percent of men who have suffered a first coronary attack could return to their original occupation" but that the coronary patient must learn to live "with moderation in his diet, exercise, and the 'drive' under which he worked," and then related that Sir Thomas Lewis, a British doctor, died with his fifth coronary at the age of 65, having had his first one when he was about 50.

We would like to see Dr. Andrus, as well as all our other health authorities, emphasize moderation in diet, exercise and the drive under which people work before a coronary attack develops, for the fact that so many come through to suffer subsequent attacks does not save those who succumb to it in the first instance.

Prevention Best

We cannot but commend the effort that is being made to counteract unreasoning fear, but the best way to accomplish this is not by pointing out that many of those who have heart attacks recover, but by following a program of living which protects us against the onset of these attacks. James Reston[11] very wisely pointed out that while many recover, many others do not, and quoted Dr. Henry Kirkland, Chief Medical Director of the Prudential Life Insurance Company, who in a paper on "Prognosis in Heart Disease," read last May, only four months before President Eisenhower's attack, stated:

"The occurrence of a documented acute coronary episode is of extremely serious moment. Sudden death is frequent. Death within a few months is common. It is only when the patient enters the third year that his chances of survival tend to brighten appreciably. . . . "

Dr. Ancel Keys, Director, Laboratory of Physiological Hygiene, University of Minnesota, dealing with the same subject, pointed out that several thousand Americans had heart attacks on September 24, 1955, the day President

---

[10] *New York Times,* October 22, 1955.
[11] *New York Times,* January 8, 1956.

Eisenhower was stricken, and that the President was merely one of the lucky ones, for "close to a thousand of his fellow citizens died of coronary heart disease that day."

"And it was a below average day. In recent years, the average daily toll from coronary deaths in the United States is considerably over 1000," Dr. Keys continued.[12]

Furthermore, there is no reason why we should resign ourselves to the idea that a coronary attack at about fifty, or even sixty-five, is a normal expectation, for the right diet, correct eating habits and moderation in living can keep our heart and arteries young and healthy even in the seventies and eighties.

That this disease does not show up suddenly but develops gradually over a period of time can be seen from our findings on the Korean battlefields, where the heart and coronary arteries of a number of young men who were killed in battle were analyzed. In "one series of 300 cases in which the average age was 22 years, the incidence of diseased coronary arteries was 77.3 per cent."[13]

The New York Times, on October 20, 1955, reported that one of our leading film actors, age forty-one, "succumbed instantaneously of a coronary thrombosis" while shaving, and that his family physician stated that the actor "had been in good health and had no history of a heart condition."

Whenever confronted by a statement of this kind, it is well to reflect on the statement by Dr. White who pointed out that a coronary thrombosis usually does not develop suddenly but builds up over a period of years.

This is true even though the attack occurs most unexpectedly, and even though the degenerative changes have not been recognized by either patient or doctor.

Increase Merely Part of a General Pattern

A point which must never be overlooked is the fact that the last half century has seen a vast growth in many

---

[12] *The Miami Herald,* February 12, 1956.

[13] Major Gen'l Dan C. Ogle, "What Air Force Is Doing to Ease Heart Risks," *U. S. News & World Report,* October 14, 1955.

of our chronic and degenerative diseases, and that the increase in the incidence of the diseases of the heart and blood vessels is merely part and parcel of this general increase.

Taking cancer as an example, we find that "while death from this disease at the turn of the century amounted to not more than three percent of all deaths, the number has risen to the point where there is hardly any country with less than eight percent."[14]

As far as the United States is concerned, while 1901 showed a cancer mortality of 66.4 per 100,000 population, the number has increased to 138.7 per 100,000 population, or more than double.

How Children's Lives Have Been Saved

That the over-all life span of man has increased in the last fifty years is undeniable. We have seen, however, that the increase has resulted primarily from a saving in children's and infants' lives and practically none at all or to a very minimal degree from a prolongation of the life of the older population.

How this saving in children's and infants' lives has come about should be of interest. An examination of the facts will disclose that the majority of deaths among our children and infants up to and during the early part of the century resulted primarily from such serious diseases as tuberculosis, typhoid fever, dysentery and pneumonia.

With the turn of the century, however, a significant reduction in the number of these diseases began to take place. The reason for this reduction has aroused some interesting discussions. Some have tried to credit our newly discovered drugs with this reduction, but it should not take much to see how fallacious this is since a significant reduction in these diseases began to manifest itself with the turn of the century, long before the introduction of these drugs. Most of our health authorities realize that extensive improvements in sanitation and hygiene, improved feeding practices, and general advances in our standard of living were primarily responsible for this

[14] From Report of United Nations World Health Organization, *New York Times*, July 16, 1952.

change. Better housing conditions, a growing appreciation of the benefits of the outdoors, as well as a sounder nutritional approach, have contributed materially to improved child health and have brought about a reduction in these serious diseases among our children.

This fact was recognized by the Metropolitan Life Insurance Company, when in their bulletin, "A Century of Progress in Longevity," they stated that the increase in the expectation of life at birth resulted because "we now enjoy a vastly higher standard of living—more abundant and better food, shelter, clothing, education and recreational facilities."[15]

The New York Times, commenting on the report of the Brookings Institution, while mentioning that credit should be given to some of the newer drugs, nevertheless, mentioned that, "Better housing, better nutrition, more time for outdoor recreation are the direct consequences of the general prosperity that the country has enjoyed off and on in the last half-century; and these have certainly conduced to better health and well-being."[16]

That progress in hygiene and sanitation, an improved nutritional regimen, and advances in our standard of living have contributed materially to the improvement in the health of our children is unquestionable. Who doesn't remember the slum conditions which existed only thirty to forty years ago? It is not difficult to recall the relatively recent time when many parents kept the windows of their homes tightly shut for fear that their children might "catch cold."

Then again, was it not only comparatively recent when the main foods in a child's diet, in addition to milk, were mostly made up of refined cereals, and white flour and white sugar products? Whole wheat bread and whole grain cereals were practically unknown in the average household, while fruits and vegetables were rarely, if ever, used.

Today most of this is considerably changed. While slum areas still exist in some of our large cities, the over-all improvements in housing conditions, and our higher standard of living, plus the general improvement in hygiene and sanitation have eradicated most of the so-called

---

[15] "A Century of Progress in Longevity," Vol. 30, Oct. 1949.
[16] *New York Times* Editorial, August 1952.

"infectious" diseases in children, and have contributed materially to the saving of infants' and children's lives.

People of all classes and walks of life are now aware that fresh air and sunshine are beneficial to health, and most parents realize the value of fresh fruits and vegetables.

Furthermore, we know that in many homes, the use of white sugar and white flour products has been substantially reduced or even completely eliminated, and that the sweet fruits, raw sugar, honey, whole wheat bread and the whole grain cereals have been substituted in their stead.

Adult Population Also Benefited

That the many revolutionary changes of the last half century have also benefited our adult population should be apparent. The tremendous strides in housing, the progress in sanitation and hygiene, the advances in nutrition, and the higher standard of living have done much to improve the comfort and well-being of our adult population.

Among the other factors which have contributed to their well-being can be mentioned our vast technological and sociological advances, which improved working conditions and reduced the hours of labor, providing more time for play, relaxation and cultural pursuits.

It is, therefore, all the more depressing when we realize that in spite of these advances, the life span of our adult population has shown only a nominal increase, if any at all, while the many degenerative diseases have continued to multiply at a tremendous rate.

We fully agree with I. J. Rodale,[17] Editor of *Prevention*, a monthly devoted to health, who stated:

"His (man's) body is ravaged by disease just as much as ever, in spite of the unconvincing mortality statisticians who, by their quirky, higher mathematics, measure death instead of health, who juggle day-old babies into the death averages," and then concluded:

"I am fifty-four and am no longer a day-old babe. I want a mortality statistic tailored to my own needs and not to that of a baby."

---

[17] *Prevention*, July 1952.

Our aim should not be to offer an excuse for the existence of these conditions, but to discover what the causes are and make an effort to correct them.

Cholesterol Makes Its Appearance

Some years ago authorities thought that they were beginning to see daylight when they discovered that people who were suffering from hardening of the arteries accumulated an excessive amount of cholesterol, a substance of fatty origin, in their blood, and that when this substance was deposited within the confines of the arteries, it caused sores or lesions, which were followed by hardening of the arteries.

Cholesterol is found in large quantities in the fatty foods of animal origin such as eggs, milk, butter, cream, as well as the fatty meats and fish. It seemed logical to assume that by controlling the intake of these foods hardening of the arteries could be eliminated or greatly lessened.

However, many of our authorities were not satisfied with this assumption. Although they were aware that a restriction in the intake of the cholesterol-rich foods benefited their patients, they were still confronted by questions which seemed baffling. For one thing, they noticed that many people who consumed large quantities of the cholesterol-rich foods did not suffer from hardening of the arteries; for another, further research disclosed that not all types of cholesterol, but only a special type, the "giant cell cholesterol," caused the damage.

Finally, they began to realize that hardening of the arteries does not develop merely from an intake of the cholesterol-rich foods but from a faulty utilization of these foods.

Research at many of our institutions confirmed this fact. *The U. S. News & World Report,*[18] a national weekly published in Washington, D. C., reported on the work done by scientists in different institutions, including the Heart Institute of the National Institute of Health in Washington, which proved that certain key substances

[18] *U. S. News & World Report,* June 13, 1952.

(hormones) which normally break up our fat foods are lacking in persons suffering from these diseases. It further stated that our scientists are now working feverishly in the hope of discovering the missing element or elements, so that where necessary, they could be supplied to sufferers from these diseases, "artificially by pill or by injection."

William S. Gailmor, discussing this subject, referred to the work of Dr. William D. Kountz of the Washington University of Medicine, St. Louis, Mo., who basing his work on the fundamental research of Dr. Timothy Leary of Tufts University, and the so-called "anoxemia" (lack of oxygen) theory of Dr. Wilhelm C. Hueper, President of the American Society of Arteriosclerosis, conclusively demonstrated that "a thyroid hormone deficiency by preventing metabolism or absorption of a fatty substance (cholesterol) into the tissues, allows it to accumulate in the arteries, ultimately causing the characteristic 'hardening.'"[19]

Stephen M. Spencer, in an article in *The Saturday Evening Post,* referred to the work of Dr. John Gofman, who in conjunction with his teammates at the Donner Laboratory of the University of California, demonstrated that "just as diabetics cannot handle sugar, so according to this theory, certain people cannot handle their butter and eggs as efficiently as the rest of us can."[20]

In short, the main factor is not merely how much of the cholesterol-rich foods we eat but how the body is able to utilize these foods.

That the excessive accumulation of cholesterol in the blood is due to an impairment of metabolism and is only one of the many changes which occur in the body as a result of this impairment is now being recognized to an ever greater extent.

Waldemar D. Kaempffert, Science Editor of the *New York Times,* referring to the work of Drs. Alfred Steiner, Forest E. Kendall, and James Q. L. Mathers of the Goldwater Memorial Hospital and the Department of Medicine, College of Physicians and Surgeons, Columbia

[19] *Daily Compass,* June 6, 1952.
[20] "Are You Eating Your Way to Arteriosclerosis," Oct. 21, 1950.

University, which proved that the two principal fatty components of the blood-cholesterol and phospholipids occur in patients who had suffered coronary thrombosis (closure of a coronary artery by a clot) but that the cholesterol in these cases increased at a more rapid rate than the phospholipids, mentioned that the relative level of phospholipids and cholesterol may be as important in the development of arteriosclerosis as the increase in the level of cholesterol itself.[21]

Dr. Meyer Friedman, Dr. Ray Rosenman, and Dr. Sanford Byers of the Harold Brunn Institute of Mt. Zion Hospital, also challenging the idea that cholesterol is the cause of arteriosclerosis, mentioned that while it was thought that cholesterol caused an increase in phospholipids, research at the Brunn Institute disclosed that the increase in phospholipids "precedes and causes an increase in cholesterol" and as such "cholesterol is an effect, not a cause."[22]

"Deposits of cholesterol, a fatty alcohol, on the walls of the arteries, are not the primary cause of hardening of the arteries. First comes mucoid proteins, then cholesterol, and large globules of fat—sometimes," is another report by Waldemar D. Kaempffert, referring to the work of Drs. Henry D. Moon and James F. Rinehart of the University of California School of Medicine.

"Moon and Rinehart saw cases of arterio-sclerosis where there were no cholesterol deposits at all—only these mucoid proteins," Waldemar D. Kaempffert continued.

Drs. Moon and Rinehart[23] did not overlook the presence of cholesterol deposits in these cases; they were merely not convinced that the cholesterol was the primary cause of the hardening.

They came to this conclusion by checking parts of arteries of people who died suddenly, some from heart attacks, other from other causes. Altogether they checked samples of arteries of 250 people ranging in age from four months to 90 years, and observed that the early changes in arteriosclerosis, especially in the coronary ves-

21 *New York Times,* June 10, 1951.
22 *New York Times,* February 14, 1956.
23 *Time,* December 1, 1952.

sels of youngsters, showed a slight thickening of the innermost layer of the arteries which was marked by an increase in deposits of muco-protein, by fibrous growths, and by breaks in the elastic tissue fibres, but no deposits of cholesterol.

The second, or later stage showed further accumulation of muco-protein, the formation of hard, fibrous plaques in the walls of the arteries and the presence of fat, and only sometimes cholesterol.

In the more advanced stages of arteriosclerosis, part of the arteries were hard and glossy looking, and deposits of large globules of fat (including cholesterol), and frequent deposits of calcium existed, causing a narrowing of the arterial tube, slowing down the flow of the blood, and exposing the patient to the danger of the formation of fatal clots.

From all this, Drs. Moon and Rinehart concluded that "fat metabolism becomes important only in the later stages of the disease and that the original trouble probably lies in how the body uses protein."

Time Magazine,[24] in reporting a talk on hardening of the arteries by Dr. Alfred Steiner, before the Pan American Medical Association, stated that Dr. Steiner "did not go into the question of what comes first, the fatty artery clogging cholesterol or the disease. Neither did he bother with the arguments as to just which abnormalities involving fatty substances in the blood are more important," but stated that "probably all play a role in the development of arteriosclerosis."

We are stressing all this to show that by pin-pointing only one of the many changes which occur as part of the metabolic disorder, we fail to obtain a true picture of what actually takes place.

It should not be difficult for us to agree with Dr. Herman T. Blumenthal[25] of the St. Louis Jewish Hospital who concluded that "hardening of the arteries may not be one disease but many" and that even the "metabolic changes which have received so much attention, may be the *result* rather than the cause of the aging and hardening of the arteries."

[24] *Time,* February 1, 1954.
[25] *Time,* December 14, 1953.

The primary objective should be to obtain a clear picture of the many facets which contribute to the breakdown in metabolism and lead to the onset of these diseases, since only in this way can we understand how this condition can be counteracted or prevented.

How We Can Assure Optimum Metabolism

One point is gradually emerging out of the welter of confusion which has been existing for a long time—namely, that if any progress is to be made in the prevention or correction of the diseases of the heart and blood vessels, the factors which lead to a disordered metabolism must be clearly understood so that they can be effectively counteracted.

The Effects of Hormone Therapy

In discussing the work of the scientists at the Heart Institution of the National Institute of Health in Washington, we pointed out that they are now trying to discover the hormone or group of hormones missing in sufferers from these diseases in the hope that they could be supplied "artificially by pill or injection."

We wish it were as simple as that! An examination of hormone therapy in other metabolic diseases such as diabetes, arthritis, etc., reveals how ineffective this type of therapy can be.

Insulin and Diabetes

Who does not remember the excitement when insulin was originally introduced? Here, we were told, was at last the solution to the diabetic problem! Now, nearly half a century later, we know that diabetes is still very much of a problem and even a greater one than it has ever been. Of even greater significance is the fact that not only does insulin fail to solve the problem of the diabetic, but in many instances it actually aggravates the problem since its use often converts a simple or incipient diabetic condition into a more serious or chronic one.

The observations of Dr. Michael Somogyi[26] and his associates at the Jewish Hospital of St. Louis, Mo., are of interest at this point. In a report made public before the American Chemical Society, Dr. Somogyi pointed out that a study of 4,000 diabetic cases conducted by him and his associates over a period of fourteen years, revealed that virtually all adult victims of diabetes can be restored to normal health without insulin injections, and that "even the less than 1% of the adult diabetics who still require insulin can get along with 20 units a day or less instead of 50 to as high as 150 units daily now taken by a large number of diabetic victims under present methods of treatment."

Dr. Somogyi then continued by asserting that when insulin is used in doses which lower the sugar below normal, it actually increases the severity of the disease, because it creates what he calls, a state of "chronic insulin poisoning."

This happens because "large doses of insulin lead to unbalancing of the delicately adjusted glandular system, particularly the pituitary gland at the base of the skull and the cortex of the adrenal gland above the kidneys."

"These glands work in unison, along with the insulin-secreting pancreas, to maintain the blood-sugar level on an even keel. When too much insulin is given, it leads to a lowering of the blood sugar to a level below normal. This, in turn, activates the pituitary-adrenal system to elevate the blood sugar back to normal," Dr. Somogyi continued, and then stated:

"The patient whose body is the scene of such a tug-of-war, becomes a severe diabetic, a victim of a form of poisoning in which insulin, administered to reduce the blood-sugar level, indirectly but inevitably raises it."

Cortisone and ACTH

Our recent experiences with cortisone and ACTH have demonstrated even to a more spectacular degree the failure of this type of therapy. Who doesn't remember the sensational reports when cortisone and ACTH were introduced only a few short years ago? And who doesn't remember

[26] *New York Times*, September 19, 1949.

the renewed hopes raised in the hearts of countless unfortunate arthritis sufferers, when the "miraculous" effects of these new remedies were first reported?

It didn't take long, however, before we began to realize that these remedies failed to live up to their original promises. Not only were they in many instances followed by side effects which were extremely dangerous, but the relief obtained from their use proved to be of only a transitory nature. As soon as the medication was discontinued, the original condition often recurred even in a more severe form.

No wonder Waldemar Kaempffert, Science Editor of the *New York Times*, wrote the following in connection with this drug:

"Whenever a new drug is discovered with astonishing properties, cautious and skeptical physicians wonder whether the benefits that follow its administration may not be accompanied by evils worse than the affliction itself."[27]

And then, a few months later, he stated: "Though both cortisone and ACTH are still more precious than radium and therefore not in general use, it is this department's prediction that both are on the way out so far as arthritis is concerned . . . some of the leading pharmaceutical houses are of the same opinion."[28]

While cortisone and ACTH are still extensively employed in a great variety of diseases, serious observers realize that their effects at best are only of a transitory nature and often lead to great harm. The findings of Doctors R. H. Freyberg, C. H. Traeger, Patterson W. Squires, C. H. Adams and C. Stevenson, conclusively demonstrated this fact.

In a report published in the *Journal of the American Medical Association*, these eminent authorities pointed out that while "in many patients a good partial suppression of the disease can be maintained on 75 mg. or less of cortisone acetate, orally, daily . . . We have been very disappointed in the post-cortisone events. Relapse in 83% of patients, including those with arthritis of less than six months duration, even after treatment for as long as a

27 *New York Times*, October 2, 1949.
28 *New York Times*, February 6, 1950.

year; severe 'withdrawal syndrome'; difficult post-cortisone readjustment to the worsened state of arthritis . . .

"There is no evidence that the course of the arthritis is ultimately altered favorably by prolonged cortisone therapy as we used it," these authors continued, and then concluded:

"Whenever cortisone is employed, troublesome effects must be expected in some patients, and the physician should be prepared to meet them."[29]

Dr. Russell L. Cecil,[30] National Medical Director of the Arthritis and Rheumatism Foundation, also acknowledged the limitations and dangers of these remedies. In an interview by William Kitay, Dr. Cecil stated:

"Like insulin in diabetes, these two hormones (cortisone and ACTH) must be continually given to maintain the desired benefits. When discontinued, relapse will occur in most cases.

"Unfortunately, a considerable number of arthritics cannot take these hormones for any length of time without developing unpleasant and sometimes severe side effects," Dr. Cecil continued further.

An interesting commentary on the value of cortisone has come to us from a New York physician whose son, suffering from rheumatoid arthritis, turned to us for help after having used this drug for some time. While, for obvious reasons, we are omitting the name of the physician, the letter containing this commentary is in our possession and can be produced on request.

In his letter, dated January 30, 1955, the physician wrote as follows:

"Since I visited you at Orlando, I have met Dr. —————— who is a fellow of the College of Physicians and an assistant professor under Dr. Hench, discoverer of cortisone and ACTH, and I told him of —————'s condition, and he heartily approved of your treatments, etc., as he stated to me, *we are disappointed with cortisone and ACTH.*" (Emphasis ours.)

[29] "Problems of Prolonged Cortisone Treatment for Rheumatoid Arthritis," December 15, 1951.
[30] *New York Herald Tribune*, "The Truth About Arthritis," December 5, 1954.

Dr. Floyd S. Daft,[31] Director of the National Institute of Arthritis and Metabolic Diseases of the U. S. Public Health Service, in his explanation why new drugs are being sought for the treatment of arthritis, stated that while these drugs (cortisone and ACTH) offered the best treatment until last August, they "can cause the body to retain salt and water . . . that puts a strain on the heart and kidneys. They can cause a puffing of the face, 'moon face.' They can cause unwanted facial hair to grow, particularly in women."

Selye[32] explained why cortisone and ACTH can ultimately lead to serious damage. He mentioned that these remedies were introduced in the belief that they would imitate what the body normally attempts to do under stress, namely, "imitate the counter-shock phenomena," but that it was later found that the increased secretion of cortisone or ACTH resulting from stress or the supply of these substances in medicinal form, can in itself become the cause of disease. He then proceeded to name hypertension, arteriosclerosis, diabetes, gout, myocarditis, and various rheumatic allergic conditions as some of the diseases that may develop.

Discovery of Hormone Likely

We have pointed out before that many scientists working on this problem are endeavoring to discover the hormone or group of hormones presumably missing in diseases of the heart and blood vessels, so that they may be supplied "by pill or injection."

It is likely that before long a particular hormone, or group of hormones involved in these diseases may be discovered and like insulin in diabetes, or cortisone and ACTH in arthritis, will be obtainable in the form of a pill or injection.

Furthermore, just as insulin in diabetes or cortisone and ACTH in arthritis, this new remedy may provide a certain measure of relief. It should, however, be evident that just as in diabetes and arthritis, the relief would be only of a temporary nature, since only when the underlying causes

[31] *N. S. News & World* Report, June 3, 1955.
[32] Selye, *Stress*, Vol. 1.

of disease are removed or checked can thorough results be obtained.

For permanent and real correction, the factors which contribute to a breakdown or distortion of metabolism must be removed or corrected, and only such care as helps to restore normal function can be of value. These changes cannot be brought about through the supply of a particular hormone or set of hormones, but through the removal or correction of all the influences which cause deficiencies, impair the functions of the glands and create a chemical imbalance in the organism.

Even where the breakdown is already far advanced and complete correction is no longer possible, it is still imperative that these changes be instituted, since only a program which removes the destructive influences and promotes rebuilding will arrest the progress of the disease and restore a measure of health and well-being.

Merely a Link in the Chain

From all that we have stated before, it should be clear that the heart and blood vessels are but part and parcel of the whole organism, and that the same causes which bring about their impairment simultaneously affect the body as a whole. In other words, the damage which shows up in the heart and blood vessels is merely a link in the chain of bodily derangements.

These influences usually operate over a long period of time and usually affect the other organs and functions of the body long before the heart and blood vessels begin to break down.

Furthermore, these abuses are usually cumulative in effect, and while the initial damage may, at first, not be apparent or recognizable, their ultimate effects are inevitable.

We have pointed out that these diseases are caused by toxins which originate within our body or which are taken into our system with food and drink, or in the form of drugs or chemicals. Tobacco, alcohol, the concentrated and processed foods, an excess of sweets, spices and condiments, overeating, strained and frayed nerves, and various harrying emotional conflicts, as well as the health-sapping and exhausting tempo of present day living, all contribute to a depletion of our energies, upset the chemical balance of the body, and give rise to the diseases of metabolism, the diseases of the heart and blood vessels included.

Low Blood Pressure

While high blood pressure is of greatest concern, it is well to mention that low blood pressure too must not be neglected since this also may be a warning that our health is not in best condition.

Low blood pressure may result from extreme debility, weakened arteries, a bad heart, an impoverished blood supply, poor quality of the blood, or a disorder of the glandular system. While it is not well known, a stroke or coronary thrombosis or other abnormal clotting phenomena could develop in cases of low blood pressure, and may result from a weakened heart or a poor circulatory condition.

The question as to whether the blood pressure is high or low can be determined in many instances only when all the factors related to it are taken into consideration. We have pointed out before that blood pressure does not have to rise with age and that a person of seventy can have as normal a blood pressure as one of twenty.

It is also well to remember that the range of blood pressure is subject to variation depending upon influences which affect the heart and nervous system and that a blood pressure of 90/60 is often found in people of normal health.

Another point worth stressing is that blood pressure is often influenced to a considerable degree by the food we eat. Rich, spicy foods often increase blood pressure, while a simple bland diet will often show a reduction in blood pressure of about 15 to 20 points within a few days, and this is actually a healthier and more normal blood pressure.

However, a rapid drop in blood pressure coupled with a weak pulse, must be carefully investigated since it could indicate heart muscle damage or weakness.

While an abnormally low blood pressure can temporarily be elevated with certain medicines or treatments, it should be apparent that only when the underlying weaknesses or disorders are overcome or brought under control can the condition be permanently corrected or improved.

CHAPTER VII

THE ROLE OF NUTRITION

That nutrition plays an important role in the treatment of the diseases of the heart and blood vessels is now well known. That unwholesome or careless nutritional habits contribute to the development of these diseases is, however, unfortunately not yet fully recognized.

While some authorities in their approach to these diseases stress the importance of limiting the cholesterol-rich foods, such as eggs, butter, milk, cream, cheese and the fat meats and fish, and while many exclude the use of salt and others restrict the intake of protein, it is essential to point out that these modifications are only a few of the changes which must be made if we are to obtain optimum results.

The nutritional habits of most people are greatly deficient. The diet of the average individual includes the use of refined and denatured foods such as white flour and white sugar products, an excessive intake of starches and sweets in the form of cakes, pastries, ice cream, etc., a large consumption of rich concentrated foods such as fat and processed cheeses, fat meats, sauces, etc.; the use of stimulants such as alcohol, coffee, tea, chocolate, as well as other beverages and foods of a stimulating nature, and the use of highly spiced or seasoned foods. These foods overtax the digestive organs, cause the accumulation of toxins in the system, and give rise to many metabolic perversions which ultimately manifest themselves in diseases of one form or another.

To restore good health, an all-around healthful, well balanced nutritional regimen is imperative.

Such a program embodies the use of simple natural

foods such as the raw and stewed fruits, raw, steamed and baked vegetables, plus moderate amounts of easily digestible proteins and carbohydrates.

It excludes the use of refined and denatured foods, controls the intake of sweets, restricts the consumption of rich and highly concentrated foods, and eliminates the use of sharp and irritating spices and condiments, as well as coffee, tea and all other stimulants.

Why Fat Foods Should Be Excluded

The reason for limiting the use of eggs, cream, butter, milk and fat meats and fish, as well as other cholesterol-rich foods should be clear. However, a point worth stressing is that even fatty foods of vegetable origin such as nuts, avocado, and the various oils, must be used in moderate quantities or even entirely omitted until results have been attained. All fat foods are difficult to digest, and as a result can impair the heart and the blood vessels.

Why Table Salt Should Be Excluded

Table salt is excluded in heart disease, hardening of the arteries, high blood pressure, and in the diseases of the kidneys, because sodium, one of the elements of table salt, is eliminated through the kidneys and can be a burden to them.

Furthermore, when the kidneys are damaged or weakened, they are unable to eliminate all the sodium, and when retained in the body, it often causes the accumulation of fluid.

Some authorities insist that even the foods which contain sodium in organic forms, as in fruits and vegetables, should be excluded from the diet. This is not only unnecessary, but may, in the long run, be actually harmful since it deprives the body of many valuable nutritional elements. The authorities who exclude the sodium-containing foods fail to realize that many of the sodium-containing foods are essential for good nutrition while table salt is not a food but a load on the kidneys.

On the Question of Protein

The question of protein has been the subject of controversy for a long time. While currently many doctors are stressing the intake of large quantities of protein, this is contrary to the findings of some of our most outstanding nutrition authorities.

Sherman of Columbia, Hindhede of Denmark, Chittenden of Yale, Clive McCay of Johns Hopkins, to name only a few of our world renowned authorities, have proved conclusively that the intake of an excessive amount of protein can do great harm to the body.

Denmark During World War I

Some of our observations during World Wars I and II have demonstrated this fact. Denmark during World War I is a case in point. The Danish people at that time were not self-sufficient and had to import part of their food supply from other countries. A blockade by the Allies made it impossible for them to import the food they needed, and a severe drought made the situation even more critical.

To cope with this problem, the Danish government under the enlightened guidance of Dr. Michael Hindhede, their Minister of Health, embarked upon a program which involved a considerable reduction in their livestock and the conversion of all arable lands to the raising of grains and vegetables. While this program reduced the available meat supply to a mere trifle, it not only saved the Danish people from the threatened famine, but also helped improve the health of the nation. Such diseases as diabetes, heart disease, arthritis, as well as many of the other chronic and degenerative diseases were significantly reduced during that period, and the general level of health was raised considerably.

Harold Westergaard, Professor of the Copenhagen University, in his English summary of the report[1] dealing

[1] Beretning Til Indenrigsministeriet om Rationeringens Indvirkning Paa Sundhedstilstanden ved M. Hindhede.

with this period, pointed out that while "the average death during the last five years before the war was, for the whole of the country, 12.9 per mille . . . the death rate during the first year of restriction from October 1, 1917, to October 1, 1918 had only been 10.4 per mille," and then concluded by stating that "never in any European country had there been such a low death rate."

In another part of the report, Professor Westergaard pointed out that whereas in Copenhagen "during the five most favorable years before the war, 1910-14, the yearly number of deaths for persons over twenty-five was 4543 (2205 men and 2338 women), the number of deaths in the year of restrictions was lower by 1016 (665 and 351) than it would have been, in case the death rate had been the same as 1910-14, or in other words, a decrease of 30 percent for men and 15 percent for women."

In all fairness to the subject, we wish to point out that this phenomenal improvement resulted not merely from a restriction in the consumption of meat, but from a complete readjustment in the living habits of the population which, according to Professor Westergaard, embraced among other things:

"1. A reduction of the quantity of protein, generally speaking, but in particular of animal protein in favor of vegetable protein.

"2. A large reduction of the consumption of fat.

"3. A very large reduction of the consumption of alcohol.

"4. A general reduction of the quantity of food."

Great Britain and World War II

The more recent experiences of the British people during World War II, one of the most difficult periods in their history, also illustrates this point. We know that the meat rations of the English during World War II were drastically reduced. Yet despite the grueling difficulties experienced by them during that harrowing period, the health of the English people not only was maintained, but actually improved.

To illustrate how meager the meat rations of the English were during the war, it should be sufficient to mention that Ernest O. Hauser, in an article in the *Saturday Evening Post,* pointed out that even as recently as January 1951, the *weekly* meat ration in England was eleven cents worth per person, and that a year later it was raised to the grand total of sixteen cents worth per week.

Two eggs and one ounce of cheese a week were the only other concentrated protein foods allowed. Yet "in spite of rationing," Mr. Hauser reports, "physicians claim that the English people are healthier than ever."[2]

Mr. Hauser's observations are in line with the statement of Sir Wilson Jameson, Chief Medical Officer of the Health Ministry of Great Britain, who stated "that the general health of this country (England) showed an improvement despite nearly four years of war" and emphasized that "one important factor in this improvement, was the simple but excellent diet imposed by the exigencies of war."[3]

In view of this authoritative statement, we wonder whether it would not have been more exact for Mr. Hauser to state that the English people were healthier *because* of food rationing and not *in spite* of it.

Our Experiences During the War Years

Our own experiences during those fateful years were also illuminating. Most of us still remember the long queues in front of meat shops, and the disappointments of many of our people when they were unable to obtain a sufficient supply of meat for their table. Due to its high cost, many people were forced to go without meat altogether, while those who could afford the high prices were able to purchase only small quantities of it. Yet, not one was any the worse off.

It was during those years that our government as well as many of our scientists pointed out that the protein we need for complete nourishment could be obtained from foods other than meat, and that we could be well nourished even if meat were completely omitted from our diet. *The*

[2] "It's No Fun To Be An Englishman," July 5, 1952.
[3] *New York Times.*

Journal of the American Medical Association declared that "Dietary protein derived in proportions of one half to two thirds from plant origin is entirely adequate in quality to meet all protein needs for normal growth, development, reproduction and lactation,"[4] while Howard B. Lewis, of the Department of Biological Chemistry, Medical School, University of Michigan, in the September 18, 1948 issue of the *Journal* stated that "both animal and vegetable foodstuffs are good sources of protein, provided that they supply adequate amounts of the essential amino acids."

This is in line with the statement of Dr. Theodore R. Van Dellen who at an earlier date stated that "since the substances in meat are not superior to those of milk, eggs, and cheese, we do not need to worry so long as dairy products are available."[5]

It was during those years that the so-called Oxford experiments were released proving that a diet containing fifty grams of protein provides ample protein and that of this amount only ten to fifteen percent of the so-called complete protein, obtainable in meat, eggs, cheese, or milk, was necessary.

A fact which is often overlooked is that the green leafy vegetables such as spinach, green peas, string beans, kale, broccoli, supply the finest type of complete protein, although not in concentrated form.

Our lowly potato also offers a fine type of easily digestible protein, although in small quantities.

While the protein foods are the tissue building materials and, therefore, essential to life, an excess can easily cause a great deal of harm. Protein is essential for growth and for the replenishment of the worn out tissues. Adults need it primarily to replace wear and tear. While starches and sugars can be stored up in the body in the form of fat, our body is not equipped to store up protein. It can use only what it needs and the excess must be eliminated. Most of it is eliminated through the colon, where, when the intake is excessive, it undergoes putrefactive changes and is capaable of creating a host of harmful waste products.

[4] "Nutritional Contributions of Wheat," November 27, 1948.
[5] "Now You Don't Have To Eat Meat; Study Your Protein!" *Daily News,* October 25, 1946.

The Value of the Non-Meat Regimen

Bogomoletz,[6] whose longevity serum, as we have seen, has proven a complete failure, nevertheless was right when he stated that, if meat is used, it be used sparingly.

"Although meat is predominantly protein foodstuff, it is also responsible for the formation of waste products that are not only unwholesome but even harmful, when functions of the liver and kidneys are impaired," he stated.

Lautman, too, pointed out that meat gives rise to harmful waste products. In his discussion of meat soups and beef broths, he stated: ". . . Soup is actually a concentrated essence of meat, low in protein substance, but rich in extractives. Since it contains only those elements of the meat which are supposed to be harmful, without retaining any of the qualities of the protein, soup as a regular article of diet would not be especially helpful."[7]

The Classical Rice Diet

In recent years the use of the rice diet in the treatment of diseases of the heart and blood pressure has gained considerable attention.

This diet, originally introduced in 1940 by Dr. W. Kempner at Duke University School of Medicine, demonstrated anew the value of a modified nutritional program. Dr. Kempner discovered this diet when he observed that the people living in countries where rice is the main staple of food had a low incidence of heart and blood vessel diseases.

This diet is very simple. The main food is rice cooked in plain water or fruit juice, with the addition of some fruit.

Spectacular results have been obtained with this diet. A marked drop in blood pressure, a reduction in the size of the heart, absorption of hemorrhages in the eye, a change in the reading of the electro-cardiogram, and a

[6] *The Prolongation of Life.*
[7] Maurice F. Lautman, *Arthritis and Rheumatic Disease.*

clearing up of edema or swellings, were some of the changes observed following its use.

A point which should be stressed is that the phenomenal benefits derived from this diet result not because of any special quality inherent in rice, but because of the limitations which are imposed in connection with the diet.

The classical rice diet eliminates the use of all salt, reduces the fat intake to no more than five grams a day, restricts the use of protein to twenty grams a day, and provides a total food intake of no more than 2000 calories per day. Furthermore, it excludes most of the so-called conventional foods, the spices and the stimulants which overtax digestion, lead to the formation of irritating toxins and are conducive to damage to the heart, the arteries, and the kidneys.

These restrictions are the real factors which contribute to the improvements in heart and circulatory diseases, and it is imperative that we recognize this fact if continuous healthful results are really desired. The sufferer from these diseases needs a suitable diet, worked out to satisfy his permanent needs, and not one which serves merely as a temporary expedient.

The rice diet itself presents many disadvantages which precludes its use for more than short periods of time. One of its disadvantages is its extreme monotony. Another is the exclusion of many fruits and vegetables merely because of their sodium content. While it is true that table salt can be extremely harmful in these cases and therefore must be excluded, this does not hold true with regard to fruits and vegetables which contain sodium. The element sodium is essential to health and it is well to bear in mind that the sodium in fruits and vegetables affects the body quite differently from the sodium present in concentrated form in irritating table salt.

While those who prescribe the classical rice diet try to guard against deficiencies by the addition of concentrated "supplements," it is well to bear in mind that the vitamins and minerals obtained in supplements can never take the place of the vitamins and minerals obtainable in food in their natural form.

One of the major fallacies of the rice diet is that it fails to take into consideration the need for an all around flexible nutritional program, and that as a result, many of its followers sooner or later return to most of their original harmful habits of eating.

Other Nutritional Requirements

While it is imperative that the necessity of a rounded, well-balanced nutritional program be recognized, Dr. Kempner deserves credit nevertheless for making large sections of the medical profession acutely aware of the importance of a modified dietary regimen in these cases. In his "Radical Dietary Treatment of Hypertensive and Arteriosclerotic Vascular Disease, Heart and Kidney Disease, and Vascular Retinopathy," Dr. Kempner stated that while in the past he advocated the use of the rice diet in all serious heart, artery and kidney diseases which did not "respond to the customary treatment with salt restriction and drugs" and in all uncomplicated cases where "a more liberal regimen has failed," he now recognizes that "treatment should be more aggressive and uncompromising and should be started as soon as the diagnosis is certain."[8]

He continued further by stating that "loss of time is as unjustifiable as it would be in cancer or tuberculosis, and the inconveniences involved are no excuse for delaying optimal dietary treatment until the more unpleasant and often irreversible complications have appeared."

We fully subscribe to this statement, and because we are also concerned with prevention, we emphasize a careful dietary program before any of these diseases show up.

Complete Nutritional Program Essential

While we enthusiastically subscribe to the modifications inherent in the rice diet, such as the restriction or exclusion of the cholesterol and other fat containing foods, the elimination of table salt, the reduction in the intake of protein, and the limitation in the total amount of food eaten, these are only some of the steps which must be taken if maximum and lasting benefits are to be attained.

[8] *G.P.*, March 1954.

For optimum, as well as permanent results, we must plan a nutritional program which includes a liberal supply of the protective foods such as raw and steamed vegetables, raw and stewed fruits, plus a moderate use of easily digestible proteins and starches, and which excludes refined and processed foods, as well as foods of a stimulating and irritating nature. A diet worked out along these lines can give us meals of a most enjoyable nature, and at the same time provide all the health and body building benefits on a much more prolonged basis.

That nutrition plays a vital role in diseases of the heart and blood vessels is now universally recognized. When Drs. Otto Saphir and Leonard Ohringer,[9] of Michael Reese Hospital, Chicago, Ill., mentioned that diet may be responsible for the increase in heart disease "in persons younger than 50," they had in mind primarily the large increase in the consumption of fat in the American diet. However it is imperative to realize that if we are really to do an effective job, all factors which enter into the formation of a wholesome nutritional program must be taken into consideration. This involves not only the use of foods which are easily digestible and which provide optimum value from the standpoint of health, but also the drastic elimination of the denatured and processed foods, as well as those foods which are difficult to digest.

Vegetables and fruits are replete in the elements which enrich the blood and build a strong and healthy body. They are most valuable when uncooked. However those who for one reason or another cannot eat them in their raw state should prepare them in such a way that only a minimum of the valuable protective elements such as the vitamins, minerals and enzymes, be lost. They may be steamed or baked but should not be fried or overcooked. In addition, no irritating spices or condiments should be added.

Another point worth bearing in mind in prescribing a well-balanced, healthful diet is that when too many foods are eaten at one meal, overeating is certain to take place and the digestion becomes overtaxed.

---

[9] *Orlando Sentinel*, April 8, 1955.

Uncooked Foods Superior in Health-Giving Qualities

Uncooked foods are living foods, foods which in addition to their easily digested protein and easily digestible carbohydrates are also a rich source of the valuable minerals, vitamins and enzymes. When because of ill health or a weakened digestion our body cannot handle uncooked foods and cooked foods must of necessity be used, we must not be content with the relief which we obtain at the moment, but must make sure that we gradually build up our health so that we can again handle uncooked foods without discomfort, since only then will we be sure that our health has been completely restored.

Dr. Pottenger's Feeding Experiment

Dr. Pottenger's feeding experiments with cats, subsequently tried on rats, "to determine the effect of heat-treated foods upon growth and development" is of interest at this point.[10]

The experiments were prompted because of the steady mortality among the cats which were used at the Pottenger Sanitarium to perform "adrenalectomies for the purpose of standardizing adrenal cortical material." The animals which were used for these experiments were fed the meat scraps from the sanitarium, together with raw milk and cod liver oil, but proved "poor operative risks although the technique was good."

In time, the sanitarium had more cats than they were able to feed, and to supply the food needs of the extra cats, they "placed an order for raw meat scraps at the market where the sanitarium meat was bought." These scraps included muscle, bone and viscera, and were fed each day to the same cats.

Before very long, a phenomenal change in the health of the cats became noticeable. "Within a very short time,

[10] Francis M. Pottenger, Jr., "The Effect of Heat Processed Foods and Metabolized Vitamin D Milk on the Dento-Facial Structures of Experimental Animals," *American Journal of Orthodontics & Oral Surgery,* August 1946.

the cats in those pens (those fed on raw meat scraps) survived the operations, the unoperated cats appeared in better health, and the kittens born were vigorous," Dr. Pottenger stated, and then continued:

"The contrast in apparent health between the cats in the pens fed on raw meat scraps and those fed on the cooked meat scraps was so startling that we decided to do a feeding experiment."

This experiment was conducted over a period of ten years on approximately nine hundred cats. All cats were fed alike, except that one group of cats was fed cooked meat while the other group was kept exclusively on raw meat. Both groups were fed 2/3 meat, 1/3 raw milk, plus cod-liver oil.

The results were dramatic. "The cats receiving raw meat and raw milk reproduced in homogeneity from one generation to the next. Abortion was uncommon . . . and the mother cats nursed their young in a normal manner. The cats in these pens had good resistance to vermin, infections and parasites.

"They possessed excellent equilibrium; they behaved in a predictable manner. Their organic development was complete and functioned normally," Dr. Pottenger stated.

Cats receiving the cooked meat scraps presented an entirely different picture. These cats "reproduced a heterogeneous strain of kittens, each kitten of the litter being different in skeletal pattern. Abortion in these cats was common, running about 25 percent in the first generation to about 70 percent in the second generation. Deliveries were in general difficult, many cats dying in labor. Mortality rates of the kittens were high, frequently due to the failure of the mother to lactate. The kittens were often too frail to nurse. At times the mother would steadily decline in health following the birth of the kittens, dying from some obscure tissue exhaustion about three months after delivery. Others experienced increasing difficulty with subsequent pregnancies. Some failed to become pregnant."

"Cooked-meat fed cats were irritable. The females were dangerous to handle, occasionally viciously biting the keeper. The males were more docile often to the point of being unaggressive. Sex interest was slack or perverted. Vermin and intestinal parasites abounded. Skin lesions and allergies were frequent being progressively worse from one generation to the next."

Pneumonia, empyema, diarrhoea, osteomyelitis, cardiac lesions, hyperopia and myopia (eye diseases), thyroid diseases, nephritis, orchitis, oophoritis, hepatitis (liver inflammation), paralysis, meningitis, cystitis (bladder inflammation), arthritis, and many other degenerative diseases "familiar in human medicine," took a heavy toll among these cats.

Unhealthy conditions of mouth and teeth, degenerative skeletal changes and malalignment of teeth were found in most of them.

"In autopsy, cooked-meat females frequently presented the picture of ovarian atrophy and uterine congestion, whereas the males often showed failure in the development of active spermatogenesis." The bones of these cats showed "evidence of less calcium" and they generally showed signs of shriveling or wasting or became overly fat with distended abdomens.

"In the third generation of cooked-meat fed animals, some of the bones became as soft as rubber and a true condition of osteogenesis imperfecta (imperfect bone structure from birth) was present," Dr. Pottenger reported, and then, at another part of the report pointed out that "of the cats maintained entirely on the cooked-meat diet, with raw milk, the kittens of the third generation were so degenerated that none of them survived the sixth month of life, thereby terminating the strain."

When these experiments were later repeated on rats, essentially the same results were obtained.

An interesting point in connection with these experiments is the fact that when raw metabolized vitamin D milk, pasteurized milk, evaporated milk or sweetened condensed milk, was substituted for the plain raw milk, bony disorders and deficiencies began to manifest themselves. Most marked deficiencies, however, occurred in the cats fed sweetened condensed milk, and Dr. Pottenger believed "that the excessive carbohydrate in the milk was responsible for much of this heavy damage."

"What vital elements were destroyed in the heat processing of the food fed the cats?" Dr. Pottenger asked, and then replied:

"The precise factors are not known. Ordinary cooking precipitates proteins rendering them less easily digested. Probably certain albuminoids and globulins are physiologically destroyed. All tissue enzymes are heat labile and would be materially reduced or destroyed. Vitamin C and some members of the B Complex are injured by the process of cooking . . . Minerals are rendered less soluble by altering their physicochemical state.

"It is possible that the alteration of the physicochemical state of the foods may be all that is necessary to render them imperfect foods for the maintenance of health. It is our impression that the denaturing of protein by heat is one factor responsible," Dr. Pottenger stated further, and then continued:

"The principles of growth and development are easily altered by heat and oxidation, which kill living cells at every stage of the life process from the soil through the plant, and through the animal. Change is not only shown in the immediate generation, but as a germ plasm injury which manifests itself in subsequent generations of plants and animals."

Dr. Jacob M. Leavitt summed up the situation very succinctly when he stated, "Living food contains an element which we have not as yet been able to crystallize. There is more to food than calories, enzymes and vitamins. There is a living energy, a form of solar energy which is not available to us except as we obtain it through viable or vital foods in their uncooked state," and then went on to illustrate what he meant by stating that "when a piece of coal is burned, it gives up a few gases and calories but when properly broken up or disintegrated can unlock untold and unforeseen nuclear powers."

While the nutritional value of uncooked food is vastly superior to cooked food, it is well to repeat that in certain digestive or nervous disorders, the patient may not be able to handle uncooked foods. When this is the case, we must make sure that the food is prepared in such a way that only a minimum of the valuable protective elements be lost. Our main objective, in these cases, however, should be to overcome the affliction so that uncooked foods can again be used without difficulty.

Nutrition a Major Factor in Disease

That the ultimate conquest of disease lies in the building of sound health through proper nutrition and not in an increase in the number of doctors and medical facilities was the conclusion arrived at, at a symposium of the New York County Medical Society.

"The ultimate conquest of our sickness and death rate does not lie primarily in the development of better medical facilities and wider distribution of physicians and dentists but rather in the development of robust health and energy through proper nutrition," was the declaration of Dr. Harold B. Davidson,[11] President of the New York County Medical Society, at this symposium.

That nutrition is a major factor in the control of our chronic and degenerative diseases and plays a vital role in diseases of the heart and circulation can be seen from the report presented by Dr. Charles Glen King,[12] Professor of Chemistry, Columbia University, and Scientific Director of the Nutrition Foundation, to the New York State Joint Legislative Committee on Problems of the Aging.

In this report, Dr. King pointed out that investigations carried on at the University of Toronto, Duke University, University of California, University of Missouri, Harvard University, the University of Wisconsin, and the University of Oslo (Norway), have clearly demonstrated "how quickly and sometimes irreversibly the body may be injured, either as a result of nutritional deficiencies, or by an excess of calories at critical periods of development," and that an "apparently mild transition deficiency (in earlier years) had set going degenerative changes in the liver, kidneys and arteries that later resulted in hardening of the arteries, high blood pressure, enlarged heart and shortened life span.

"One cannot attribute all of the top-ranking diseases to malnutrition as a sole cause, but nearly all research men do agree that nutrition plays an important, and often a dominant, role in all of them.

[11] *New York Times*, May 7, 1948.
[12] "Food For Later Years," *1953 Yearbook of N. Y. State Joint Legislative Committee on Problems of the Aging* (Enriching The Years).

"It is national tragedy to let the present faulty eating situation continue, when the corrective measure—simple good food, but less total food is so simple to learn and so advantageous to apply," Dr. King concluded.

Rockefeller Foundation Experiments

That faulty nutrition plays a major role in the production of many of our diseases has been demonstrated by some of our most outstanding investigators. Dr. Victor G. Heiser, of the Rockefeller Foundation, in a talk before the American Association for the Advancement of Science,[13] pointed out that large scale animal feeding experiments in India, in which the diets eaten by various sections of India's millions of people were fed to large colonies of animals reproduced, at the will of the research workers, the same state of health and well-being, and the same types of disease observed in the human population," and then continued:

"Among the parts of the body which developed various types of serious diseases in the animals fed the faulty diet were the chest, ear, nose, upper respiratory passages, the eye, gastrointestinal and urinary tract. The skin, blood, lymph and glands, nerves, heart and teeth.

"The diseases included stomach ulcers and two cases of cancer of the stomach, sinusitis, adenoids, inflammations of the eye, infections of the middle ear, pneumonia and bronchiectasis, loss of hair, skin diseases, pernicious anemia, seven types of diseases of the kidney and bladder including several types of kidney stones, goiter, enlarged adrenal glands, polyneuritis, various types of heart disease and even mal-occlusion of the teeth and a large percentage of tooth decay.

"On the other hand, the animals getting the diet eaten by some of the people of northern India developed no illness of any kind for two and a half years, corresponding to forty to fifty years in the life of man. Furthermore, none died during that period from natural causes . . . and there was no infant mortality," Dr. Heiser emphasized.

[13] "Big Feeding Tests Give Disease Clue," *New York Times,* June 21, 1939.

Now what were the diets which produced such varied results?

"This health diet, eaten by the animals and the human beings in some parts of northern India, consisted of whole wheat flour, unleavened bread lightly smeared with fresh butter, sprouted Bengal gram (legume), fresh raw carrots and cabbage ad libitum, unboiled whole milk, a small ration of raw meat with bones, once a week, and an abundance of water for drinking and washing purposes," Dr. Heiser stated, and then continued:

"The ill-balanced diet fed to the animals that developed the thirty-nine varieties of diseases common among the human beings eating the same type of food consisted mostly of cereal grains, vegetables fats, with little or no milk or butter or fresh vegetables."

The experiments by Dr. Pottenger, the large scale investigations carried on by the Rockefeller Foundation, and research carried on at many of our universities, have conclusively demonstrated the importance of nutrition in the prevention and control of heart and blood vessel diseases.

They also proved the superior value of uncooked foods over cooked foods and have amply demonstrated the importance of including a liberal amount of raw fruits and raw vegetables in our diet, proving furthermore the superiority of natural, unrefined food products over refined denatured foods.

So far as the findings of Drs. Pottenger and Heiser in relation to meat are concerned, we do not wish to imply that meat be eaten raw, but their findings are clear. If meat be eaten, it is best eaten raw.

We have seen before that meat is really not an essential food since the finest type of protein can be obtained from the vegetable and dairy products. However, if you feel that you must have meat, our advice is that only small quantities of it be eaten and that it be supplemented with a plentiful supply of raw fruits and vegetables.

The Importance of Small Meals

Next to knowing what to eat is the question of how much to eat. We have pointed out before that small meals are now considered a "must" in cases of heart disease. Dr. King's statement that we should eat "simple good food, but less total food" if we wish to stay well and live a long life, deserves special emphasis.

James Rorty in "The Thin Rats Bury The Fat Rats" pointed out that studies conducted over a period of twenty-five years by Clive McCay and associates at Cornell University, demonstrated "that it is possible to double the normal life span of the rat; to delay the onset of the degenerative diseases that rats—and human beings—normally die of . . . simply by keeping . . . on an excellent diet which is low in calories . . . "[14]

It should be clear why this is so important in diseases of the heart and blood vessels. Large meals overburden the digestion and this in turn overtaxes the heart, while small meals lessen the work of the heart and help in more rapid recovery.

Next to eating small meals, other habits of eating need watching. We must make sure not to eat too fast, chew our food thoroughly, eat only when hungry, and not eat when mentally disturbed or emotionally upset, for all this militates against good health.

The Importance of Preparing Food Properly

The importance of proper food preparation also needs stressing. Overcooked and fried foods lose most of their protective and many of their nourishing values. What have we gained when, while preparing vitamin and mineral rich fruits and vegetables, all or most of their valuable protective and nourishing elements are leached out or destroyed?

Reviewing the change in the food habits of our population, we are aware that the consumption of valuable fruits and vegetables has materially increased in the last forty years. However, because of our failure to use many of these foods in their natural state, and because of incorrect methods of preparation, many of their valuable elements are destroyed and lost, and as a result we fail to obtain all possible value.

[14] *Harpers Magazine,* May 1949.

We have seen that while phenomenal benefits are obtained from the so-called "rice" diet, these benefits result primarily from the elimination of salt, the avoidance of fats, a restriction in the intake of protein, and an over-all reduction in the amount of food eaten. However, because of its monotony, patients usually adhere to this diet only for limited periods of time and then drift back to their former eating habits. We offer our plan of eating not merely as a temporary makeshift but as an extended program of living because of its superior and lasting results.

Some people hesitate to adopt our way of eating on the assumption that our meals also may be dull and monotonous. This is not at all the case. Our meals can be made not only nutritionally satisfying but also most enjoyable.

We urge the elimination of refined and denatured foods and the exclusion of highly concentrated foods, but what a variety of savory foods we offer in their stead! All the fresh fruits, luscious berries, and melons in season, all the vegetables prepared in a hundred different ways to bring out their most delicate flavors, and the many whole grain products which are so much more delectable than those baked or prepared from white, processed flour, provide a variety of foods which make each meal a pleasure.

At this moment much is being written about the effects of fat foods, the need of restricting the use of salt in heart cases, the benefits of a rice diet, and the importance of limiting the total food intake. While all these factors are important it should be apparent that really to guard against the onset of any of these diseases, or, for that matter, against any disease of a chronic or degenerative nature, the importance of an all-around wholesome, nutritional program must be stressed. It seems to us that Dr. Charles Glen King[15] was right when he stated that "it is utterly foolish to emphasize too greatly the role of only one or a few nutrients, such as a single mineral, sugar, protein or vitamin, or the nutrition of a single part of the body, such as the hair and the skin," and then continued by saying that "that is why nutrition scientists

---

[15] "Research in Nutrition Confirms Need for Balanced Meals," Robert K. Plumb, *New York Times,* January 8, 1956.

are so heartily in agreement with us in believing that the only reasonable goal in nutrition is a lifetime concept of good food habits."

Normal Bowel Function

Many who suffer from heart and blood vessel diseases are constipated or afflicted with some digestive or intestinal disorder. Too much food or eating too fast will cause excessive gas formation even under normal conditions, and the gases pressing upward against the heart will cause considerable discomfort.

Where the digestion is already impaired, the tendency to gas formation is only intensified, and in cases of heart disease, can be extremely dangerous.

The Benefits Derived From the Omission of Food

"I saw few die of hunger . . . of eating, a hundred thousand," said Benjamin Franklin.

We cannot stress too strongly the benefits derived from small meals. In line with this, complete abstinence from food for limited periods of time in some cases can be even more beneficial. When food is eliminated for a day or two or even longer, our organs of digestion are given a chance to rest, while the kidneys as well as all other organs of elimination are able to catch up with their work of eliminating the accumulated toxins from the system. The experiments reported by Cutter and the benefits derived from the Karrell diet (mentioned in another part of this book) illustrate how effective such therapy can be.

This does not mean that one can abstain from food indiscriminately or resort to this procedure in a haphazard manner. It must be carefully supervised and should not be extended beyond the point physiologically advisable in the individual case.

A point worth stressing in connection with total abstinence from food is that, except where an emergency exists, the patient should be properly prepared for it, physiologically as well as psychologically.

A change to a better diet and a tapering off to less food, plus plenty of sleep and rest, are advisable for a few days or even longer before a fast is undertaken. A program of this kind can be highly beneficial not only in case of disease but also as a measure of prevention.

However, it is important to bear in mind that while such a regimen can be highly beneficial, its benefits can be quickly dissipated by a return to a conventional way of eating or by overeating.

CHAPTER VIII

THE LIFE ENDANGERING CHEMICALS AND FOOD ADDITIVES

The necessity of avoiding all chemically preserved foods or foods to which chemicals have been added cannot be stressed too strongly.

The era in which we live has rightly been called the era of chemistry. The chemical industry has grown by leaps and bounds, influencing our existence in many ways. Practically every industry is dependent upon it and the food industry is no exception.

However while its contributions to industry as a whole have been of tremendous value, its use in the food industry has turned out to be a menace to health and life.

Congressman James J. Delaney, Chairman of the Non-Partisan House Selective Committee to Investigate the Use of Food Products, pointed out that 704 chemicals are now being used in the food industry "of which 428 are known to be safe."[1]

"In other words," Congressman Delaney pointed out, "276 are unknown and untested, and some of them may be slowly poisoning us!"

Some of our past experiences strongly support Congressman Delaney's conclusion. It was not so very long ago when the papers were filled with the story of "agene" (nitrogen trichloride),[2] a chemical used to bleach the flour used in the baking of our bread and cakes. Research workers suddenly discovered that when this chemical was

[1] "Peril on Your Food Shelf," *American Magazine*, July 1952.

[2] "Agene Toxicity," Silver, Johnson, Kark, Klein, Monahan & Zevin; also other reports in *JAMA*, November 22, 1947.

fed to animals, it induced various nervous reactions including fits of an epileptic-like nature, and it was as a result of these findings that the Food and Drug Administration finally prohibited its use.

Agene had been in use in the baking industry as a flour bleaching agent for over a quarter of a century, and 95 percent of all breads and cakes sold commercially were prepared from flour containing this chemical. Although some of our foremost nutritionists kept warning us against the use of this chemical, the baking industry continued to use it without restraint until recently, and discontinued it only when it was banned by the Food and Drug Administration.

We cannot help wondering how many cases of heart disease or other diseases of a degenerative nature may have had their inception or may have become intensified as a result of this dangerous chemical.

Not too long afterward, another chemical, lithium chloride, used as a salt substitute in cases of heart and kidney diseases and high blood pressure, was found injurious to health and was ordered withdrawn from use.

Fortunately lithium chloride was not in use for very long, but even for the short time that it was used, a number of fatalities was reported.[3]

Recently a group of chemicals used as bread softeners in the baking industry—the polyoxyethylene monostearate and related compounds, were ordered discontinued by the Food and Drug Administration.

In ordering that the use of these chemicals be discontinued, the Food and Drug Administration explained that the ban became necessary because these chemicals "could deceive consumers as to the age of the bread—and because they had not been tested adequately for their safety as ingredients of bread."[4]

Another reason, according to Commissioner Charles W. Crawford of the Food and Drug Administration, was that "these compounds were derived in part from ethylene oxide, a stranger in the food world."

---

[3] "Lithium Poisoning from the Use of Salt Substitute," Corcoran, Taylor and Page. *Journal of the American Medical Association,* March 12, 1949.
[4] *New York Times,* May 15, 1952.

Let us be grateful for small favors. However, while being grateful for the discontinuance of these chemicals, one cannot but wonder why similar and probably equally questionable bread softeners are still being permitted.

From the report of the Food and Drug Administration, it is apparent "that about 80% of all bread and rolls manufactured commercially contain emulsifiers (bread softeners)" and that only about 1/3 of the bread and rolls baked commercially were affected by this ruling. Since one of the reasons for the prohibition of the use of the polyoxyethylene monostearate and related compounds was because they "could deceive consumers as to the age of the bread," in what way are the other emulsifiers, still in use in about 2/3 of the bread and cakes baked commercially, any less deceiving?

Furthermore, does the fact that the other emulsifiers are still being permitted mean that they have been found to be harmless, or must we, as in "agene," wait a quarter of a century before the detrimental effects of these chemicals are recognized and steps are taken to outlaw them?

Dr. Robert Riley,[5] Director of the State of Maryland, Department of Health, in a report presented at the 97th annual convention of the American Medical Association, referred to a number of chemicals which are being used in bread and cakes baked commercially. Among them he mentioned "potassium bromate which is used to make the flour easier to handle and produce loaves of greater volume," also sodium bicarbonate, calcium phosphate and sodium acid pyrophosphate, each used for a different purpose. While some of these chemicals, according to Dr. Riley, may be harmless or innocuous, what tests have been made to determine their long-range effects? Furthermore, is their use any less deceiving?

The Danger of Chemical Pesticides

That the arsenical sprays used in agriculture are harmful has been known for a long time, but unfortunately

[5] "The Health Dept. and The Food of The People," *Journal of the American Medical Association,* Oct. 2, 1948.

nothing so far has been done to prohibit their use. As a matter of fact, the use of these compounds has grown tremendously in the past thirty years, and Dr. Riley points out that "the danger to the consumer (of receiving a toxic amount of arsenic) is thus constantly increasing."

While Dr. Riley is hopeful that "insecticides free from toxicity to human beings will in time replace the present dangerous substance," the insecticides introduced most recently, according to recent health investigators, are actually even more dangerous.

We can think back to the time when, many years ago, Alfred W. McCann, Sr., in the *New York Globe,* conducted his one-man crusade against the use of these dangerous sprays, and when Dr. I. Sirovich, then Congressman from New York, in a series of articles published in the *Daily Mirror,* emphasized the harmful effects of these chemicals. Since then, the use of these chemicals has become only much more widespread and nothing is being done to discontinue their use.

Congressman Delaney referred to the synthetic hormone STILBESTROL which is used by poultry breeders "to add weight quickly and increase the market value of their products," and pointed out that in Canada its use has been outlawed because it can lead to sterility in the young.

A point which is often overlooked in connection with this hormone is that it is seriously suspected as a carcinogenic (cancer producing) agent.

With regard to phosphoric acid, a chemical used by the soft drink industry, Congressman Delaney referred to the experiments at the Naval Medical Research Institute which "have shown that a human tooth put in soft drinks containing phosphoric acid lost its enamel and became soft in 24 hours."

DDT is now being used extensively as an insecticide and fungicide in and around barns. Congressman Delaney mentioned that DDT accumulates in the body fat of the animal and gets into our bodies through the meat we eat, and that this "can eventually have a cumulative and serious effect on the liver."

He continued further "that people suffering last winter from Virus X exhibited the same set of symptoms as those suffering from DDT poisoning."

Chlordane, an insecticide introduced in 1947 and now used extensively on fruits and vegetables, is, according to the statement of Dr. A. J. Lehman, Director of Food and Drug Administration's Pharmacology Division, "four or five times more poisonous than DDT."

In a report published in the *Journal of the American Medical Association,* Dr. O. Bruce Lemmon and Commander Wilmot F. Pierce stated that their investigations disclosed that "continuous administration of chlordane to laboratory animals caused focal hepatic necrosis (liver degeneration), edema (swelling), congestion and exudates in the lungs and degenerative changes in intestinal submucosa and in the convoluted tubules of the kidneys."[6]

Dealing with the same subject, Dr. Paul Lensky and Dr. Howard Evans in the same issue of the *Journal*[7] described a case of poisoning of a fifteen-month-old child due to accidental swallowing of "probably not more than a mouthful" of a mild chlordane solution, and stated that "the insecticide enters the body by absorption through the intact skin, by inhalation of dusts or sprays, and by ingestion."

U. S. News & World Report reported that the Committee on Pesticides of the American Medical Association issued "a fresh warning against the dangers of poisoning through improper use and careless handling of chlordane. . . . "It cautions against using chlordane in areas frequented by children, in waxes and polishes that touch the skin and slow liberation of fumes—especially in closed, heated rooms."[8]

One can well understand why Dr. Lehman stated that he "would hesitate to eat any food that had any chlordane residue on it."

Congressman Delaney reflected on the "growing number of mental diseases" and wondered "if there is not some connection between the increase in mental diseases and the many new chemicals used in our foods."

We too have often wondered about this, and in addition have also wondered how much of a connection there is between the increase in the diseases of the heart and blood

6 "Intoxication Due to Chlordane," *JAMA,* August 2, 1952.
7 "Human Poisoning by Chlordane," *JAMA,* August 2, 1952.
8 "News You Can Use," September 2, 1955.

vessels as well as the many other chronic and degenerative diseases and the use of these chemicals in our foods.

We have seen from our experiences with "agene," lithium chloride, and other chemicals, as well as from the facts elicited by Congressman Delaney of the Non-Partisan House Select Committee, how dangerous some of these chemicals can be, and we cannot refrain from asking, why are there no steps being taken to check the use of these dangerous chemicals?

In explaining the reason for their use in food processing, Congressman Delaney tersely stated that "they are relatively cheap, easy, and work 'wonders' as preservers, blenders, softeners, bleachers, emulsifiers, insect and fungus killers, and crop stimulators."

While the food industry is quite adamant about its right to use chemicals in the manufacture of its products until or unless they are proved harmful, it should be evident that the only way to serve the interests of the public is to establish rigid controls and not permit the use of any chemical in the food industry before its long range effects have been fully tested and evaluated.

The immediate question, so far as the consumer is concerned, is what can we do to protect ourselves against this mass danger? For one thing, we urge that whenever possible, packaged and manufactured foods be avoided, since many of these foods are processed and contain chemical preservatives.

Where such foods are used, it is important that all the printed matter on the label, including the small print, be carefully read to find out what has been added. While the law requires that all ingredients be listed on the label, the chemicals and preservatives which are added are usually printed in the smallest type, often barely legible to the naked eye.

In an endeavor to avoid the use of foods which have been grown with chemical fertilizers, or which have been chemically treated or sprayed, some of our health conscious people are turning to the use of organically grown fruits and vegetables. These foods grown on soil which is organically fertilized and without the use of chemical conditioners or the various chemical pesticides or insecticides, are infinitely richer in taste, flavor, and quality. We urge our readers to become more familiar with this type of farming, and whenever possible use the fruits and vegetables that are grown this way.

Those who raise fruits and vegetables organically employ special farming methods which help them put back into the soil in organic form and not through the addition of chemicals, the elements which are taken out of it. This type of farming keeps the soil properly conditioned and enables it to maintain its own immunity against the insects and pests which otherwise menace the crop.

Natural Immunity

This is very much in line with the immunity which exists in the body when we are in a healthy state. It is well known that our best protection against dangerous bacteria and viruses and harmful foreign substances is found in the immunity of our own body, and the same holds true with regard to the soil.

The New York Times in an editorial, January 26, 1941, aptly stated that "if ever we had an abuse of science and technology, it is in the matter of preparing food for the eye rather than for the stomach. It is no credit to society that it has invoked chemistry and engineering to impoverish rather than to enrich food, and that the supposedly backward peasant of Europe, who must content himself with a crust of black but wholesome bread of his own baking and such vegetables as he himself can raise, is physically better off than our own farmers, who are as dependent on the store for canned fruits, vegetables and flour as are the workers of our industrial communities" and that "it may become necessary to control the preservation, processing and packaging of food as rigorously as we control the quality of drugs."[9]

While this was written in 1941, the situation has not materially changed, but if anything, has considerably worsened.

Dr. Pottenger pointed out that man is part of a biological cycle and that to obtain optimum health that cycle must be maintained and then showed how this cycle is broken through poor soil culture, stating that intensive

[9] "American Diet," *New York Times,* January 26, 1941.

cultivation has depleted the soil to such an extent that crops of optimum value are no longer produced and that while "mineral fertilizers have been used to make up for this depletion, they are not enough." He then went on to emphasize that organic or living fertilizers must be used to produce a fertile soil "which in turn will produce excellent crops."[10]

"The nutritional value of plant and animal products is diminished under conditions of depletion and this, in turn, decreases the biological efficiency of man," Pottenger concluded.

For those who are not in position to obtain the organically grown, insecticide free, fruits and vegetables, the use of diluted hydrochloric acid to wash off the poisonous sprays used in agriculture, is being suggested by leaders in the health field. The *Journal of the American Medical Association,* in reply to an inquiry, mentioned that one ounce of concentrated hydrochloric acid diluted with three quarts of water will remove "the commonly used inorganic insecticides such as lead arsenate, Paris green and cryolite" and "remove most of an organic insecticide such as DDT." The food washed in this solution for five minutes will do a satisfactory job of removing the residue of most, if not all, of the poisonous insecticides, according to this reply.[11]

The editor, in reply to this inquiry, also stated that "Public Law 518, passed on July 22, 1954, as an amendment to the Federal Food, Drug, and Cosmetic Act, requires that residues of pesticides on fruits and vegetables not exceed a tolerance that is regarded as safe food," but it should be apparent that this is far from providing the protection we need. For one thing, it is well known that the tolerance of individuals for chemicals and drugs varies, for another, we must always bear in mind that chemicals, as well as drugs, tend to accumulate in the body, and that as a result, their harmful effects may not show up for some time.

At this point, we wish to utter a word of warning.

---

[10] F. M. Pottenger, Jr., "The Reciprocal Relationship of the Health of Plants, Animals and Human Beings." *American Therapeutic Society Transactions,* 1941-1942.

[11] *Journal of the American Medical Association,* February 18, 1956.

While it is sound policy to use every precaution to obtain wholesome and poison free foods and to do everything possible to wash away or remove the poisonous sprays from our foods, it is extremely unwise to permit ourselves to become so panicked about the foods we eat, that we lose our balance or peace of mind.

Let us follow a sensible routine of using only the best of foods (best from the standpoint of nutrition and selection), and of preparing them in the best way possible, and then let us be content in the knowledge that we are doing everything possible to avoid the pitfalls that confront us. While we deplore the existence of this hazardous situation and while we should try to do everything we can to counteract or eliminate the harm that can arise from it, we would endanger our health only more, if we started to worry every time we sat down to eat a meal.

We know that the last word on the subject of organic agriculture has not been spoken and we realize that a great deal of work is still to be done before this subject is fully clarified. However, there should be no question that denatured and processed foods are a hazard to health and that the use of the poisonous insecticides and pesticides is a grave danger to us.

We Must Watch What We Eat

It is incomprehensible to us why some people are so adamant in their refusal to make a change in their diet even when it is obvious that it would be for their health. Some justify this attitude by pointing out that many people who have never worried about their diet lived to a ripe old age, overlooking the fact that a great many more were unable to get away with it. Furthermore, they fail to realize that in the past, people lived closer to the soil, and the refining and processing of food as well as the use of preservatives were either unknown or in their infancy.

The contrast between the simple foods of the past and the foods of today, which Weston Price called "The Foods of Commerce," from which most of the vitamins, minerals and enzymes have been removed, speaks for itself. Those who have grown up in a peasant country will recollect how vastly superior in flavor and taste are the fruits and vegetables which are grown on natural soil and under natural cultivation, and how much better they are than those which are raised with chemical fertilizers and under more intensified farming methods.

CHAPTER IX

THE SMOKING QUESTION

With all the news recently appearing in the press, no one has to be told that smoking is harmful. While recent reports dealt primarily with the effect of smoking on the lungs, its detrimental effects on the heart and circulatory system, although not as extensively publicized, have been known for a long time.

Dr. Alton Ochsner, Chairman of the Department of Surgery, Tulane University, School of Medicine, in a talk before the Greater New York Dental Society, pointed out that medical men are now "extremely concerned about the possibility that the male population of the United States will be decimated by cancer of the lung in another fifty years if cigarette smoking increases as it has in the past, unless some steps are taken to remove the cancer-producing factor in tobacco," and sardonically added:

"Smoking may have at least one virtue, by smoking heavily a man may have a heart attack: then he would not live long enough to develop lung cancer."[1]

At a recent meeting of the Public Health Cancer Association, an organization related to the American Public Health Association, where a resolution was adopted urging the discontinuance of smoking as a protection against cancer of the lungs, one participant stressed the fact that there was good reason to believe that smoking causes "cancer in body sites other than the lungs and the oral areas" while another stated "that the now suspected relationship between smoking and heart disease might

[1] "Cancer Rise Laid to Smoking," *New York Times,* December 9, 1953.

eventually prove to be more significant that the present relation between smoking and lung cancer."[2]

Dr. Theodore R. Van Dellen in one of his syndicated articles, stated that cancer of the lungs as well as smoker's throat and smoker's bronchitis is caused by the tars and other combustible materials in tobacco. He then went on to say:

"The second effect of tobacco is produced by nicotine that is absorbed into the blood as it passes through the membranes of the respiratory passageways." He then quoted Dr. Grace Roth, of the Mayo Foundation, University of Minnesota, who pointed out that 2.5 to 3 milligrams of nicotine is absorbed from the lungs from one standard cigarette and that while some individuals are more sensitive to the chemical than others, "The blood vessels suffer most; nicotine causes them to constrict."[3]

Dr. Roth, who has done a great deal of research on the effects of smoking, incidentally pointed out at the 29th annual meeting of the Greater New York Dental Society that nicotine causes an increase in blood pressure and pulse and a decrease in skin temperature and followed this up by reading a paper prepared by Dr. Irving S. Wright, of the Cornell University Medical College, which stated that "the use of tobacco may mean the difference between life and death for persons with diseases of the circulation."[4]

While Dr. Morton L. Levin, Assistant Commissioner of Medical Services of the Health Department of the State of New York, dealing specifically with the effect of smoking on the lungs stated "that the relative incidence of lung cancer among men who smoke twenty or more cigarettes a day was ten times that of non-smokers," and that "those who smoked less than one pack a day had five times as much lung cancer as non-smokers,"[5] the American Cancer Society, in its report at the annual convention of the American Medical Association, pointed out that

[2] *New York Times,* September 12, 1954.

[3] *Daily News,* November 3, 1953.

[4] "Cancer Rise Laid to Smoking," *New York Times,* December 9, 1953.

[5] "Ten Times More Lung Cancer Among Pack-a-Day Smokers," *New York Herald Tribune,* March 15, 1954.

death from all causes among the cigarette smokers was up to 75 percent higher than non-smokers.[6]

"For men smoking a pack a day the general death rate from all causes was 75 percent above that of non-smokers. For men smoking cigarettes alone, it was 63 percent higher counting all causes, but 82 percent higher for heart attacks and 106 percent higher for cancer," they stated.

Dr. Charles Cameron of New York, Medical and Scientific Director of the American Cancer Society, himself a smoker and at first reluctant to admit that smoking is harmful, could not but realize the gravity of the situation, acknowledging "that the smoking picture based on large segments of population was admittedly grim."[7]

Dr. Harry J. Johnson, head of the Life Extension Examiners, a nationwide group of physicians specializing in physical examinations for industry, only confirmed what other scientists are finally beginning to recognize. Studies covering 2,000 men disclosed that "smokers complained of cough 300 percent more often than non-smokers, of irritation of nose and throat 167 percent more often, of heart spasms 50 percent more often, of shortness of breath 140 percent more often, and of heartburn 100 percent more often."[8]

The New York Academy of Medicine, entering into the discussion on the effect of smoking, pointed out that it was well known in medical circles that moderate smokers died sooner than non-smokers and that heavier smokers had an even shorter life expectancy and then called attention to the findings of Dr. Raymond Pearl of Johns Hopkins Department of Biology who sixteen years ago disclosed that "deaths would start occurring among heavy smokers at age 35 and would continue to outnumber the deaths of non-smokers and light smokers all the way to age 70 at which time mortality rates tend to level off."[9]

The findings of Dr. Raymond Pearl were known in medical and scientific circles, and as we were reading this report from the New York Academy of Medicine, we

[6] "Cigarette Smokers Die Sooner," *New York World Telegram*, June 21, 1954.

[7] *New York Times*, June 22, 1954.

[8] *New York World Telegram*, June 26, 1954.

[9] *New York World Telegram*, June 23, 1954.

couldn't but wonder why our responsible medical organizations failed to stress this point before, and why some of them even went out of their way to minimize or deride his findings.

Why Doctors Condone Smoking

Occasionally we are asked why, if smoking is really harmful, do doctors condone it? We shall defer to Dr. Martin Gumpert[10] who has answered this question quite lucidly and unequivocally:

"It is, of course, an open secret that medical prohibition or tolerance of tobacco depends a great deal on the physician's own smoking habits," was the way Dr. Gumpert put it.

Dr. Gumpert, once a heavy smoker, was forced to give up smoking because of a heart attack. He was aware of many warning signals preceding the heart attack, but like the many others who are addicted to smoking, disregarded them. "My pulse rate had for some time been definitely higher than it should have been; yet the extra beats were merely considered by me as of no consequence, while a smoker's cough was put down as an unpleasant, but necessary evil," Dr. Gumpert stated, and then went on to say that it took a heart attack to make him realize the dangers of smoking.

Dr. Alton Ochsner only confirmed Dr. Gumpert's explanation. "Unfortunately many physicians, probably because they themselves smoke, are unwilling to admit that there is a causal relationship between smoking and cancer of the lungs, in spite of the overwhelming statistical evidence," Dr. Ochsner stated.[11]

The economical aspect also enters into the picture. The tobacco industry is an immense industry and large sections of our population depend upon it for their existence. It is evident that millions of people would suffer economically if a vast segment of our population ceased smoking.

Our government too has a financial stake in the industry. According to the *New York World Telegram,*

10 Dr. Martin Gumpert, "The Dangers of Smoking," *Tomorrow,* March or April 1934.

11 "The Case Against Smoking," *The Nation,* May 23, 1953.

taxes collected by the Federal Government from this industry amount to about $1,600,000,000 annually while the States collect an additional 488 millions yearly.

However, as Dr. E. Cuyler Hammond of the American Cancer Society so pertinently pointed out, there is much more to this question than economics, since in addition to the economic angle, our government also has "a stake in the welfare of our people, and in this instance the stake is the more than 20,000 deaths from lung cancer a year with an ever mounting toll."

While Dr. Hammond failed to mention it, in addition to the 20,000 or more deaths from cancer of the lungs, we must also think of the hundreds of thousands of deaths from heart and circulatory diseases, as well as other diseases of a degenerative nature in which smoking plays a part. We are in complete agreement with Dr. Clarence Williams Lieb, who in his book *Safer Smoking* mentioned that if he had his way every pack of cigarettes would be inscribed with "a skull and cross-bones."

That smoking disturbs the fat metabolism and raises the fat level of the blood to a point where it becomes a contributing factor in the development of heart disease has been demonstrated only recently by the work of Dr. John W. Gofman, Professor of Medical Physics at the Donner Laboratory Division of Medical Physics at the University of California in Berkeley. In the course of a research project carried on at the University of California financed by the United States Atomic Energy Commission, Dr. Gofman (in association with Dr. Frank Lindgren and Beverly Strisower, Oliver de Lalla, Frank Glazier and Arthur Tampli) demonstrated that twenty or more cigarettes increased the fat level of the blood in male subjects sufficiently "to raise the overall coronary heart disease death rate by 40 percent."[12]

While Dr. Gofman asserted that "the process by which giant particles in the blood are increased by smoking" and "the mechanism by which large fat particles (including cholesterol) contribute to heart and artery affliction" are not known, and while he recognized the fact that the "lipo-protein elevation resulting from cigarette

[12] "Cigarette Linked to Heart Disease," *New York Times,* September 6, 1955.

smoking may not be entirely responsible" for the higher incidence of coronary disease mortality, his statement that "it must account for an appreciable portion of it" was quite significant.

Smoking Not the Only Villain

While the facts that smoking is harmful are overwhelming, and while we fully agree that those who persist in smoking shorten their lives, we were nevertheless pleased to note Dr. Gofman's admission that other factors besides smoking may also be responsible for this alarming increase in mortality. This fact must be recognized if we wish to obtain a clear and comprehensive picture of the situation and really accomplish results. Without justifying the motives of those who seek to minimize the adverse effects of smoking, it is nevertheless imperative that we realize that smoking is only one of the many harmful influences which contribute to the high incidence of these diseases, and that unless all adverse factors are recognized and removed, we will fail in our efforts to remedy the situation. While we must not minimize the effects of smoking, we must also not overlook the effects of the polluted air we breathe and its evil effect upon our health. The exhaust from automobiles, the dust from the asphalt roads, the smoke-belching factory chimneys and the fumes from our coal and oil furnaces, all affect our health adversely.

Waldemar Kaempffert,[13] Science Editor of the *New York Times,* quoted Dr. Morris B. Jacobs, Director of the Laboratory of the New York Department of Air Pollution Control, and Dr. Leonard Greenberg, New York's Commissioner of Air Pollution Control, to the effect that "more than a million and a half tons of odorous, eye-smarting sulphur-dioxide gas—from which 2.2 million tons of corrosive sulphuric acid may be formed are poured into New York City's atmosphere each year" and then added that "coal and fuel oil are the chief villains in the sulphur dioxide picture, but there are numerous others such as motor vehicle exhausts, smoky incinerators, outdoor trash fires and polluted air. . . ."

---

[13] *New York Times,* October 2, 1955.

Leonard Engel in *Pageant*, April, 1955, called attention to the work of Dr. F. J. Flint who demonstrated that Cor pulmonale or "lung heart," a condition which prevents normal functioning of the lungs and interferes with the flow of blood through them, is caused by deadly air contaminants such as soot, gasoline vapor, unburned droplets of oil, and sulphur dioxide, and is responsible for many deaths in many of our industrial cities.

Furthermore, who can deny that improper food, incorrect eating and drinking habits, nervous tension, lack of poise and self control, etc. play an important role?

However, we must emphasize that the fact that other factors are also involved does not make smoking any less hazardous.

Dr. W. C. Hueper,[14] head of the Environment Cancer Section of the National Institute of Health, one of the most vocal critics of those who claim that smoking is primarily responsible for the frightening increase of cancer of the lungs, in one of his latest statements, mentioned that smoking plays, at most, a "possible contributory role" and that "atmospheric pollutants are to a great part responsible for the causation of lung cancer."

We agree with Dr. Hueper that it is wrong to stress only the factor of smoking and minimize "the widespread presence of industry-related atmospheric pollutants of recognized carcinogenic (cancer causing) properties," on the other hand it is wrong to overlook or try to minimize the fact that smoking, too, causes a pollution of our air passages and as such is a vicious health destroying habit.

Furthermore, what about the continuously increasing evidence of the detrimental effects of some of the chemicals in tobacco on the heart and the circulatory system?

How to Stop Smoking

Once you have reached the point where you realize that smoking is harmful and that it is best that you discontinue it, the question naturally arises, how to go about it. We are not going to pretend that it is always easy to break this habit. While some do it with relative ease, others find it a most exacting task.

[14] *New York Times*, January 21, 1956.

It is easy to understand why some find it more difficult than others. The more firmly an addiction is rooted, the more difficult it is to break away from it. However, we can help ourselves considerably by approaching the problem with the right point of view. To begin with, it is well to start by keeping constantly in mind the fact that smoking is harmful. When you do this, you will not feel too sorry for yourself for trying to give it up. Then, you must realize that it is a habit like any other habit, and that habits can be broken just as they can be acquired. Others have succeeded in doing it, and why shouldn't you?

A method which has helped many in overcoming this habit is well worth mentioning at this point. Modern man is enslaved by many bad habits, and it is well to keep in mind that one stimulating habit only begets another one. To conquer the habit of smoking, it would be tremendously helpful if all other stimulating habits would be discarded.

Coffee, tea, alcohol, spices and condiments, sweets, the use of white flour and white sugar products, rich sauces, all keep the body in a constant state of stimulation, each stimulant keeping awake the desire for the others. One stimulating habit often only chains us to all the others.

The experience of a man who succeeded in giving up smoking is worth relating at this point. The man was making plans to take his customary summer vacation, but this time decided to spend it at a resort where nutrition and careful living habits were stressed.

Since he was a confirmed smoker, he brought along two cartons of cigarettes and a box of cigars. "No Smoking" signs in the living and dining rooms caught his attention. To comply with this rule, he made it a practice to pick himself up after each meal and go outdoors for his habitual smoke.

This seemed a "must" to him during the first few days of his stay, but as time went on, he found that his desire to smoke became less urgent and before very long, actually dispensable. The eating of simple, unseasoned food, plus the relaxing atmosphere apparently diminished his desire to smoke and it did not take long before he lost his craving for it and gave up smoking altogether.

"It seemed natural to smoke after a steak dinner with French fried potatoes, coffee and cake; but I just had no desire for it after one of the simple vegetable meals which were served at this resort," he commented happily.

This doesn't mean that it will work as easily in all cases. People differ in temperament and will power, and the adjustment in some cases is much more difficult than in others. However, even where real difficulties exist, it must still be done if health is to be rebuilt.

Always remember that with each smoke, you only keep adding to your difficulties. Also bear in mind that there is no such thing as "can't" when we are really determined to accomplish anything. Others have done it, and so can you! Your life and health are certainly much more important than the momentary pleasure you derive from smoking. And what is even more important is that as you conquer this habit, you acquire an entirely new outlook on life and a variety of wholesome new pleasures.

In many cases, the day to day proposition has proven successful. We start this by making the patient feel that he is giving up smoking only for one day. A day later, he is urged to do it for one more day. It may seem difficult, but after all it is only one more day; and come hell or high water, he decides to stick it out! The third day comes along; well, since he has been able to do it for two days, why not one more day?

By then the sharp edges of the craving have in many cases begun to wear thin, and the person begins to realize that the battle is, after all, not as difficult as it seemed at the start.

In many cases, the confirmed smoker may, at first, become extremely restless or irritable, even as the dope addict is miserable when he is deprived of his favorite "drug." He sometimes feels as if he is ready to "jump out of his skin." This, however, wears off before long, and what joy when he finally realizes that he has conquered his enslaving habit and is now master over himself!

Once this stage is reached, it would be a serious mistake to test oneself by taking even one puff, for this may undo all the good that has been done since it can re-awaken the old craving all over again. It is like the drunkard who thinks he has overcome his addiction to liquor and then takes a drink to see whether he can "take it."

Once you have gained control over this habit, persist in carrying on, and you will be able to boast of the fact that you too have gained mastery over yourself. You can do it just as the many others have done it. Get started, be persistent, and as time goes on you will feel happy and gratified at a good deed well done!

Occasionally the craving may reassert itself even after you have reached the point where you think the habit has been completely overcome. This is a dangerous moment and you must guard against it. One careless puff and all can be lost again.

Some people insist that they are unable to stop smoking, but what they really mean is that they have not as yet made up their minds to do it.

A habit is nothing more than something we have done for so long that it has become part of us. A good habit enriches our life, while a bad habit harms us even though its potentialities for harm are not always immediately recognized. Any habit is developed by doing a certain thing constantly, a harmful habit just the same as a good habit. Replace your harmful habits by good habits and you will only be the happier for it.

Wishful Thinking

In the past, many doctors who condoned smoking maintained that no direct relationship had been found to exist between smoking and heart disease. This argument certainly does not hold water. What difference does it make whether the harm is caused directly or indirectly? Once we recognize that it is harmful, it must be eliminated. This applies with equal force to smoking, as well as to all other harmful influences or unwholesome habits of living.

Dr. Lemmon Johnson, dealing with the subject of smoking in the British Medical Journal, *Lancet,* after mentioning that "tobacco contains a number of poisons such as nicotine, pyridine bases, carbon monoxide and arsenic" went on to say that while smoking becomes "a general analgesia against life's little, or even big stresses and vexations"; in other words, while it is an escape from life's vicissitudes similar to the escape an alcoholic finds in liquor, it is hardly worth persisting in once you realize the harm it does.

Once you gain mastery over this habit, you will find an

"accession of high spirits, energy, appetite and sexual potency, with recession of coughing," Dr. Johnson pointed out.

However, before we can expect the public at large to accept this idea, doctors must set the example, Dr. Johnson said.

"About 80% of us are smokers," he estimated sadly, "and we behave collectively like an addict. Radical cure of tobacco smoking lies in its prevention and tobacco smoking is no more difficult to prevent than opium smoking. Our duty is plain."

Southwestern Medicine did not mince any words in taking doctors to task for condoning the use of tobacco. After pointing out that the nicotine in tobacco, one of the most toxic known alkaloids, increases blood pressure and pulse rate, contracts peripheral blood vessels, reduces vital capacity and gastric motility, and after stating that "it is obvious that cigarette smoking cannot but aggravate coronary heart disease and peripheral vascular disease," it then asked how, with all the evidence before us, "can we justify our own use of tobacco, or our practice of condoning the tobacco habit in our patients?"[15]

Those who persist in smoking despite all this evidence might well ponder the words of Dr. Peter J. Steincrohn[16] who stated: "When I look back over the years, and think of the thromboangiitis cases who would not give up smoking after warnings, and actually lost two legs by amputation; when I think of coronary patients who persisted in smoking two or three packages a day in spite of warning and who died prematurely, I marvel how intelligent individuals calmly go about killing themselves."

[15] "Why Do Doctors Smoke," *Southwestern Medicine,* December 1955. Reprinted in *Reader's Digest,* February 1956.
[16] *New York World Telegram,* May 9, 1953.

CHAPTER X

THE EFFECTS OF ALCOHOL

It was practically only yesterday when some doctors considered smoking a harmless pastime, while others actually encouraged it for its allegedly beneficial effects.

While the healing professions are now awakening to the dangers of smoking, this cannot be said with regard to their attitude towards liquor. Most of them still regard it as a harmless indulgence, while some even encourage it on the assumption that if used moderately, it will counteract nervous tension or help digestion. Some recommend it because it promotes a happier frame of mind and greater sociability.

We do not deny that, like smoking, liquor will produce some of these immediate effects. However, close observation will disclose that its long term effects are entirely different.

Lichtwitz pointed out that alcohol destroys the thiamine (vitamin) reserve in the liver, and that as a result, the liver is forced to take these vitamins from the nerves. The final result is that the liver "like the gastro-intestinal mucosa and the salivary glands exhibits atrophy and cellular degeneration."[1]

MacCallum declared that alcohol is "the commonest of poisons that affect human beings and that protracted habitual use seems to give rise to many anatomical changes in the organs."[2]

Henry H. Rusby asserted that "small quantities of alcohol, properly diluted taken into the stomach, produce an agreeable sensation of warmth" and hasten the diges-

[1] *Functional Pathology.*
[2] *A Textbook of Pathology.*

tion and absorption of food, but then continued to say that "the continued recourse to this artificial aid to digestion tends to necessitate it, and in increasing degree. Larger and larger amounts are apt to be required, and the natural powers of digestion become permanently and seriously impaired, and at length may be almost completely lost."[3]

He pointed out its effects are like "those of a drug which for a very brief period stimulates, then depresses the tissues upon which it acts." It is "wholly depressing" upon the nervous system, weakens the will power and the higher functions of coordination, damages the liver, frequently induces Bright's Disease, and affects the functioning of the heart and circulation.

In this book we are primarily concerned with the effects of liquor on the heart and the blood vessels.

Wassergus cited the studies of Dr. Sigmund L. Wilens, who came to the conclusion that the reason alcoholics fail to show as much arterial hardening as the non-alcoholics is because they usually die younger than non-alcoholics, or because in many cases of chronic alcoholism, alcohol takes the place of food. As a result, alcoholics are rarely obese, and therefore seldom suffer from high blood pressure, diabetes or any other condition which would predispose them to hardening of the arteries.

Wassergus concluded by stating that "if the chronic inebriate does not die of hardening of the arteries, it is usually because he doesn't live long enough."

Alcohol is often prescribed as a remedy in angina attacks because it supposedly dilates the blood vessels. Three respected research scientists, Dr. Henry I. Russek, Charles F. Naegels, and Frederick D. Regan of the U. S. Marine Hospital, Staten Island, New York,[4] pointed out that the relief obtained in angina pectoris through the use of alcohol is obtained primarily from its sedative effects and not from the dilation of the blood vessels.

However, while the "sedative effects might be good for a patient with an angina attack, it could so thoroughly mask the pain with a false sense of fitness that the patient

---

[3] *Reference Handbook of the Medical Sciences.*
[4] "No Alcohol for Angina," *Newsweek,* June 12, 1950.

would not know what ailed him until it was too late," these authorities concluded.

Alcohol is injurious not only when taken in excess, but even in small doses, and don't let anybody tell you differently!, The quarterly *Journal of Studies on Alcohol* published at Yale University[5] referred to the work of Dr. Kjell Bjerver and Dr. Leonard Goldberg (of the Department of Pharmacology of the Karolinska Institute in Stockholm) who, by testing thirty-seven skilled drivers between the ages of twenty-five and forty-five who were accustomed to drinking moderate amounts of alcohol, proved that 2-3 pints of 3.2 beer or 3 ounces of eighty-proof spirits impaired their driving ability to between 25 to 30 percent, even though they otherwise showed no obvious symptoms of intoxication.

"The usually careful drivers became careless, judgment was impaired, self-confidence and casualness were increased and they pretended not to notice the commissions of an obvious error," were some of the observations of these two noted scientists, who finally concluded that even "a small amount of alcohol causes a sharp decline in the driving ability of normally expert drivers."

That drinking and smoking complement each other and intensify the harm to the body was attested to by Dr. Sully Charles Marcel Ledermann, Chief of the section of economic studies of the French National Institute of Demographic Study, Paris, who in a report presented to the United Nations Conference on population, stated that the risks of alcohol and tobacco "seem not merely to add up but to multiply one another."[6]

In taking note of the many profound achievements of today, we cannot but wonder what greater heights of achievement we might have attained had we been free from the debilitating effects of tobacco and alcohol.

The Social Aspects of Tobacco and Alcohol

Tobacco and alcohol are accepted as part of our normal social amenities. Many people are aware of their harmful

[5] *New York Times,* March 15, 1950.
[6] *New York Times.*

effects but are unwilling to stop indulging for fear of appearing different from the others.

If you really wish to discontinue these habits, the problem is really not so difficult as it seems. You simply offer your apologies, and are done with it.

If you are fearful of offending or are unwilling to attract attention, you can do it more tactfully. If offered a cocktail, accept it graciously, if necessary even place it to your lips, but do not drink it. A cigar may be put in one's pocket "for later use."

But it really isn't too difficult to say "No, thank you" and how often people will remark, "How smart you are; I wish I could do the same!"

CHAPTER XI

THE DANGERS OF OBESITY

"One of the common complications of obesity is damage to the cardio-vascular system," stated Drs. Morris B. Green and Max Beckman,[1] and then pointed out that abnormal electro-cardiographic changes in their obese patients with hardening of the arteries were eight times as frequent as in the non-obese.

Studies carried on by the life insurance companies over an extensive period of time have proven conclusively that excess weight is not only dangerous to the heart and the vascular system (blood vessels) but also to all other vital organs of the body and is, therefore, a menace to health from every point of view .

Dr. Louis I. Dublin, Chief Statistician of the Metropolitan Life Insurance Company, in one of his recent reports on the subject mentioned that "a recent study among employees of the Metropolitan Life Insurance Company showed that elevation of the blood pressure was more than twice as frequent at ages 45 to 54 and three times as frequent at the ages of 35 to 44 among those of heavy build as among those of light build."[2]

You will notice that excess weight is considerably more dangerous in the 35 to 44 than in the 45 to 54 age groups. This is clearly in line with the greater increase in mortality from heart and vascular diseases in these age groups, and undoubtedly one of the factors which is responsible for it.

[1] "Obesity and Hypertension," *N. Y. State Journal of Medicine,* June 1, 1948.

[2] "Overweight—America's #1 Health Problem," *Today's Health,* September 1952.

"Another study based on a sample of 74,000 industrial workers showed at every age and among both men and women, a steady increase in the average blood pressure with increase in weight." Dr. Dublin continued:

"Among Army officers a group of men who were initially carefully selected and on whom careful medical observation was continued as long as they were in service, the rate of development of high blood pressure was about two and a half times as high in those who were overweight as in those who were not.

"A similar study of army officers showed that, on the average, the men who had or later developed diseases of the heart and vascular system were heavier than their fellow officers," Dr. Dublin mentioned.

"But this is only one phase of the picture and not the only penalty of overweight," Dr. Dublin stated, and then pointed out that four-fifths of those who develop diabetes after 40 are overweight, that gall bladder disease is found more frequently among the overweight, and that it is "an important contributing factor in the development of degenerative arthritis, one of the most common diseases of middle and later life."

A study by the Metropolitan Life Insurance Company covering more than 50,000 men and women, conducted over a period of twenty-five years, disclosed that the mortality from diseases of the heart and vascular system among the overweight was 50 percent higher in men and 75 percent higher in women, from gall stones more than twice as high, while from cirrhosis (hardening) of the liver, two and a half times higher, Dr. Dublin pointed out.

Dr. W. H. Sebrell, Jr., Director of the National Institute of Health (before the National Food and Nutrition Institute), is another one of the many who emphasized that obesity is the number one nutrition problem in the United States, pointing out that the "significance of this is apparent from the fact that mortality rates for the obese are well above average at every age, and rise steadily with increasing weight."[3]

James Rorty referred to the findings of life insurance companies which have proven that even as little as 10

[3] "Obesity Is Termed #1 Nutrition Ill," *New York Times*, December 9, 1952.

percent of overweight increases the mortality rate 20 percent. If you are 15 to 25 percent overweight, your chance of dying prematurely is 44 percent greater than the average.

"If you are more than 25 percent overweight, your chance of dying prematurely is 74 percent greater than that of your normal contemporaries."[4]

Dealing with the effect of overweight in cardio-vascular diseases, Rorty mentioned that life insurance companies have proven that "overweight increases the mortality by 62 percent"; and continued by quoting Dr. Stieglitz, author of *The Second Forty Years* who "believes that more than half the cases of heart exhaustion in later years are due to obesity."

Reports appearing in the *New York Times* referring to "research conducted by Professor H. C. Sherman (Columbia), Professor Clive McCay (Cornell), and others leave no doubt that if we want to live long, we must not overeat," and that a diet low in calories and high in quality of its nutritional elements, proteins, minerals and vitamins "would while keeping us thin, not only add years to life but also life to the years, postponing the slowing down processes that come past middle life and preserving the greatest resource of civilized man, his intellectual capacity, over a much longer period," should be of interest.[5]

Doctors Should Set an Example

Strange as it may seem, doctors as a class are more overweight than those in most other professions. Dr. Donald B. Armstrong, Vice-president of the Metropolitan Life Insurance Company, as well as many other physicians, stressed this fact at the convention of the American Medical Association, June 12, 1951, and belabored their obese colleagues for failing to do something about it.

Some years ago, a physician connected with one of the life insurance companies came into our office and noticing a scale in one of the corners stepped on it to weigh himself. He tipped the scale at 200 pounds.

[4] "The Thin Rats Bury the Fat Rats," *Harpers,* May 1949.
[5] " 'Longevity Diet' Told to Chemists," September 9, 1942.

"Doctor, why don't you reduce?" we asked him.

"I don't seem to be able to do it," he replied almost apologetically.

"It's simple; all you have to do is eat less."

He hemmed and hawed, and finally came up with the answer that he was working too hard and therefore "could not control his appetite."

Dr. Edward L. Bortz undoubtedly must have had some of these doctors in mind when he remarked that "we're going to have to take off the kid gloves in dealing with people who are wallowing in their own grease."

The Man Mountain—A Mountain of Flesh

One of the most interesting cases of overweight that we remember is the case of a physician who weighed about 280 to 290 pounds, and who, because of his weight, was dubbed by many of his friends as "The Man Mountain."

The first time we met him was at a restaurant. When we ordered a fruit salad, he ordered the same, but he later confessed that in all his life he would never have thought of ordering a fruit salad.

We would frequently visit patients together, and once while on a trip, we stopped the car to buy some fruit. It was one of those times when he vowed that he was again "dieting," since he was getting sicker by the day.

He too stepped out of the car, ostensibly to make a telephone call. But when he returned from the store, mustard was dripping from his lips. Evidently the telephone call was but an excuse for grabbing a "hot dog" on roll.

Once he became very ill. He could hardly breathe and his legs swelled up like a balloon. He knew that his heart and kidneys were in bad shape. We pleaded with him. "Dr. . . . . why don't you control your appetite?"

This time he pledged that from now on he would really be careful. He decided to go on a juice diet and he assured us that this time he would do a real job.

About two or three days later, he came to see us again. Because we were busy with a patient, he had to wait in the anteroom. Quite by accident, as we looked out of the window, we noticed that our good doctor was crossing the street and buying an ice cream from the "Good Humor" man who was just passing by. Somewhat later, the following dialogue took place between us:

"How is your dieting coming along?"

"Oh, fine!"

"Is ice cream part of your diet?"

He realized that we must have seen him through the window, and turning red, he mumbled, "A portion of ice cream is the equivalent of two glasses of orange juice."

This wonderful physician died at the age of 53. He was a great friend and beloved by everybody who knew him. He had a keen mind and was willing to do anything which would help his patients, but was not strong enough to conquer his own appetite and so shortened his life by many years.

Mountains of Flesh Can Melt

However, for each one who fails to do a good job, there is another one who succeeds and who benefits from it.

We can think of another case much the same as the one before. This man was twenty-eight. He wasn't really ill, he said, but he realized that he had to reduce.

We smiled when he said he wasn't ill. He was puffing and wheezing and dragging his load before him. He suffered from frequent heartburn, and a sour stomach made him very uncomfortable.

He was an accountant, and every afternoon while working over his books, he would find himself getting so drowsy that he was unable to stay awake.

He was planning to be married and he felt he owed it to his future wife to reduce. At any rate he realized that his present life was not very pleasant, and he was determined to change.

And it wasn't so hard. He watched with a sense of satisfaction the shrinking of his waistline, and he was jubilant when at last he could announce that clothes that he had to discard years back because of his increased weight were again usable and comfortable to wear.

At first he didn't think that he had been sick, but he was pleasantly surprised when, after reducing about sixty pounds, he found that his puffing and wheezing and all other abnormal symptoms had completely disappeared.

His drowsiness by then was a thing of the past. He was as alert and awake as anyone. There was a new buoyancy in his steps. And when people complimented him upon the change in his appearance, he became really proud of his accomplishment.

Eating for Two

There have been many misconceptions about weight, and the sooner these misconceptions are recognized, the better it is for all concerned.

Years back, pregnant women were under the impression that they had to eat "for two." If they wanted to stay well when pregnant and have a healthy baby, they had to eat "plenty."

Recently a man told us that when he married, his wife was a slim, petite, beautiful girl, weighing 109 pounds; but because of this mistaken idea, she permitted her weight to climb to 149 pounds during pregnancy. The more she spread out, the more of her charm and youthfulness were lost and before long, she was just an ordinary, middle-aged housewife.

This old superstition is gradually fading away, but there are still many who cling to it.

Another superstition which still lingers among many mothers is the idea that the heavier their children are, the healthier they are. This leads to constant stuffing and overfeeding, which not only makes their children fat, but also lays the foundation for many diseases.

The well-known humorist, Sam Levenson, himself rather heavy, once mentioned that his mother believed that children had to eat plenty to grow big and healthy, and that as a result his brother had become so healthy that "he couldn't even walk."

His mother, who was quite heavy herself, was persuaded at one time to go on a diet. She was quite happy at first, but couldn't overcome her fear that she might be hurting herself. She would keep looking into the mirror, repeating again and again that she was beginning to look like "skin and bones."

Many people realize that excess weight is harmful but lack the will to control their appetite, and therefore keep looking for short cuts.

Many doctors still prescribe thyroid extracts which often cause great harm, others prescribe other hormones, or laxatives of various kinds, but it is well known that none of these remedies accomplish their objective.

At the meeting of the American Medical Association, where the question of obesity arose, Dr. Stromont stated that the drug dinitrophenol, at one time used for reducing, raises body temperature so that "the obese are literally frying in their own fat."

Some believe that long walks or heavy exercises will work off their excess weight. As a matter of fact, long walks and strenuous exercises only increase the appetite and invariably induce overeating. They also overtire the body which may actually require rest rather than increased activity to rebuild normal glandular functioning.

While more rest may be necessary, this does not mean that exercise or activities are to be omitted. It merely means that we must guard against an indulgence in exercises or activities which overtire the body and weaken the functions of the glands still further.

Rest, deep breathing to increase the oxygen supply to the tissues, and moderate exercises, regulated in accordance with the need of the individual, are of great help in reducing. For permanent results, however, a well-regulated nutritional program is imperative.

If you fail to work at it our way, you are doomed to failure. You may lose a few pounds but how quickly you regain them!

And to what lengths we often go to fool ourselves! Examples like the one of the obese doctor could be cited in the thousands. Recently a man told me about a woman who was young and beautiful, but extremely overweight. She ate constantly and never knew when to stop. Finally she decided to go on a diet.

One time, while on a trip with some of her friends, she suddenly reminded herself that she had to make a telephone call. We'll never know whether she actually had to make the call, but the people who were with her in the car knew that her real reason for going into the candy store was to gulp down several pieces of candy.

Many fool themselves this way and then keep on complaining that they do not know why they are not reducing. They are just not honest with themselves. The most important factor in reducing is to eat less. Begin by cutting your food intake in half, eating very little or none of the foods you crave most. Discontinue white bread, white cereals, cakes, cookies, candy, creams of all kinds, sauces, and use more of raw and stewed fruits and raw and steamed vegetables, with small quantities of your favorite protein, once a day.

Exclude all sugars and all fat foods. Discard the use of condiments and spices. Table salt tends to put weight on by retaining fluid in the system, and should therefore be eliminated from the diet. Furthermore, do not be afraid to go without a meal or two. An eliminative regimen for a day or two, or even several days at a time, will work wonders. It will hasten the reducing process and benefit you immensely. Our task is not only to reduce weight but to rebuild the body to the point where the glands and the digestive organs function normally. After the correct weight is attained, this program of living must be continued if you are to maintain your gain or, to say it otherwise, to hold down what you have lost.

When people say that they cannot reduce, they merely mean that they haven't yet reached the point where they are willing to try hard enough. In almost all cases, results are attainable if we are willing to apply ourselves diligently to the job. The problem is merely how to go about it most efficaciously. Determination and stick-to-itiveness are the surest way to surmount the problem.

People often eat too much without realizing it. Others eat too much because they have too much time on their hands and don't know what to do with it. For some, eating is an emotional outlet.

If you have too much time on your hands, find something of interest to do to divert your mind from food. Perhaps a hobby, or some such outlet as music, literature, gardening, the outdoors, or some social interest; anything which diverts the mind and counteracts boredom is helpful.

When confronted with a problem, some fall into the habit of "compulsive" eating, but it is well to realize that not only does this not solve any problem, it adds but another one. Analyze your problem, discuss it if need be with one who may be able to advise you properly, and make the necessary adjustments. But do not seek an escape in overeating.

Some people claim that they hardly eat anything, and yet keep on gaining weight. If they would only make a list of what and how much they eat, what a surprise it would be to them! They simply do not realize how much they eat.

By following the suggestions on diet outlined in this book and by cutting down to half the quantity of food usually eaten, effective and lasting reduction will be inevitable.

And make all these changes cheerfully! Don't act the martyr and don't feel as though you are doing somebody a favor or making a great sacrifice. You are doing the only thing which will help you gain renewed health, increased strength, new vigor, and with it, a new "look," as well as an entirely new outlook on life. Aim high and do it graciously, joyously, and under your own power. Your rewards will be commensurate with your efforts.

CHAPTER XII

NERVOUS TENSION

In this world of tension, very few people know how to lead a serene and contented life. From very infancy, all through childhood and well into adulthood, we are trained to strive, to conquer, to succeed.

In business, as well as in social and cultural endeavors, we desire to excel and win acclaim, and this competitive existence leads to constant tension and ultimately becomes a permanent pattern and vicious cycle.

This is the reason so few people know how to relax or how to take life more at ease. Most people blame the increase in heart and blood vessel diseases on this high-strung, keyed-up existence, but are unwilling to recognize the fact that this type of existence can be altered. They are simply unwilling to make the changes which are necessary to alter their pattern of living. It should hardly be necessary to point out that this is an immature approach and does not solve anything.

There is no question but that nervous tension and the difficulties of our present day existence affect our health, but we delude ourselves when we place the blame exclusively on these factors and refuse to recognize the many other causes which contribute to our breakdown.

Because the majority of people are unwilling to concede that most of the influences which are responsible for their breakdown are within their control, many of them seek to shift the blame on factors for which they cannot be held responsible. To those people we would like to point out that a cursory examination will reveal that our life today is in reality much less difficult than it was in years past, and that this excuse is offered merely as a cloak to cover up an indifference or unwillingness to give up some of the unwholesome habits of living.

Who doesn't remember the depression years with their hopelessness and despair, with millions of people deprived of the very necessities of living, with nothing to look forward to? Who doesn't remember the poverty and insecurity of the sweatshop era, when people were slaving fourteen to sixteen hours a day in unhygienic, unclean workshops, and then, after work, spending the remaining few hours of the day in squalid, unsanitary tenement homes? Then, what about the war and post-war problems which took a great deal out of us?

When some of us begin talking of the "good ol' times" and start blaming the increase in many of our chronic and degenerative diseases merely on the stress and strain of present day existence, let us not forget the difficulties and hardships of the past.

When confronted by problems, it is actually a matter of self-preservation to sit back and reappraise them so that we may discern how best to deal with them. Have you ever heard of "the richest man in the cemetery?" The forty-odd year old executive who decides to slow down, even though this means doing less business, is perforce a wise man indeed. Life is too valuable to be squandered in the chase for a few more dollars or a little additional glory, nor should it be thrown away by indulging in unnecessary health-destroying habits.

Each one of us must pause and think seriously of how best to readjust our way of doing things, for no matter how close we get to our goal, whether it be in striving for wealth or in the attainment of any other possessions, if in the process of doing this our health is sacrificed, our life is a failure.

The man in his prime who is suddenly forced to give up his business because of a heart attack has managed his life poorly. Even though he has amassed a fortune or attained the pinnacle of his objective, he has failed to make the most of life. He hasn't accomplished very much, whatever his achievements, if in attaining his objective he has brought about his premature collapse.

How Life's Problems Should Be Handled

This does not mean that we should disregard our problems or be indifferent to our needs. We must learn to approach and deal with our problems with calmness and understanding, since this is the only way to cope with them adequately. Furthermore, we must make sure to follow a sound and well-regulated program of living, for only this enables us to maintain a high standard of health and endows us with the strength and vitality we need if we are to handle our problems efficiently and make life a success.

Always keep this in mind: healthy people do not succumb when confronted with a difficult problem or faced with hardships. Those who possess the stamina and endurance which goes with sound health, do not break down during periods of stress, but face their problems with equanimity and handle them in the most effective way possible. We saw typical examples of this during the depression years when millions of people were stripped of their possessions in a matter of minutes. Those with strong bodies and healthy nerves were able to take their reverses in their stride and start life all over again, while those with shattered nerves and depleted bodies were unable to bear the brunt of the burden and went to pieces altogether, often dragging their families along with them.

Emotional Problems

The points we have made regarding our every-day problems of life apply with equal force to our emotions. Tension, fear, greed, hatred, jealously, resentment, insecurity, gnaw into our vitals and destroy our heart as well as the rest of our body. Composure and self-control, on the other hand, keep us free from these harmful emotions, and protect us against their deleterious effects.

Emotional imbalance and instability are really signs of immaturity, and harm the individual who gives way to them most of all. Life cannot be fashioned in patterns of our own choosing, and when adversities arise, we must make sure that we are mentally and physically equipped to cope with them.

Calmness, composure, patience, and understanding are traits which are easily developed by the healthy person; and these qualities enable us to cope with our difficulties and help to make life a joy instead of a torment. Some people are more sensitive than others and react more keenly to their surroundings or their problems, but this need not create unhappiness. As a matter of fact, this type of temperament can actually enrich our life, provided we understand how to direct our emotions into the proper channels. People with this type of temperament possess a much greater appreciation for the things which make life more beautiful, such as the arts, literature, music, and have a great capacity for love, compassion and understanding. It is only when these sensitive qualities are misdirected or uncontrolled that they give rise to suffering.

Problems arise constantly and will continue to arise as long as we live. This is part of life and need not make life unbearable. What we must do is to develop the calmness and balance to help us handle these problems and take them in their stride. If you are one of those sensitive individuals, what a world of beauty and warmth can open up for you, provided you learn how to readjust your outlook and how to handle your problems intelligently. This may not always be easy, but many compensations will come your way, once you achieve it. Beauty, love, kindness, understanding, joy, compassion, are some of the great qualities within your reach, and are the attributes which are conducive to tranquility.

An easy way to make this adjustment is to choose a favorable time of the day when you withdraw to a quiet room, and while relaxing in a comfortable chair or in a reclining position, retrace all your actions and thoughts of the day, freely recognizing your shortcomings, and picturing how you would handle similar situations or problems in the future. After having done this, continue in your calm and relaxed position, picturing yourself as the person you would like to be, with the strength that you wish to possess, and the weaknesses that you are determined to overcome. In other words, visualize the person you wish to be, and keep on visualizing it daily until it becomes a part of you.

CHAPTER XIII

RHEUMATIC FEVER

Hard and brittle arteries or damaged kidneys ultimately lead to heart disease. Various acute diseases, too, place a strain upon the heart and often leave their imprint upon it.

One of the acute diseases which is often followed by heart damage is rheumatic fever, a disease which affects most often the young. About 75 percent of all who suffer from rheumatic fever are below the age of twenty.

This disease takes a terrific toll of human life. About 50,000 children are known to die from it yearly, and many of those who survive are left with permanently damaged hearts.

Those who recover from their first attack are always in danger of recurrent attacks, and each succeeding attack is usually of a much more serious nature.

At least one-third of all adult heart diseases arise as an aftermath of rheumatic fever, while ninety percent of all heart diseases in children are of this type.

Rheumatic fever was originally regarded as an acute rheumatic disease of the joints. However, since so many of these cases are followed by heart damage, many authorities now classify it as a disease of the heart.

E. C. Laseque once described this disease as the disease which "licks the joints and bites the heart." However, it should be of interest to mention that this disease frequently affects other parts of the body as well. The kidneys, the nerves, as well as many other parts of the body, may be affected by it. When the nerves are affected, it gives rise to the condition known as chorea, or St. Vitus Dance.

Another point worth mentioning is that in many cases

of rheumatic fever, the joints may be completely free from pain.

At this point, we wish to stress the fact that while the heart in many of these cases may be affected from the very beginning, no permanent heart damage need result from it. The type of treatment employed will often determine whether the patient is left with permanent heart damage or comes through unscathed.

The conventional treatment in rheumatic fever is rest in bed, the application of heat, plenty of "good" food, and the use of aspirin. Aspirin is regarded as a specific in this disease, and is part of the armamentarium of the average physician.

While there is no question that rest in bed and the application of heat are of great help, physicians would do well to reevaluate the effects of aspirin, as well as the conventional type of feeding, in the light of our new concepts of disease and the more modern findings of nutrition. They would soon realize that a change from the conventional approach is imperative if permanent heart damage is to be avoided.

Let us begin by examining how aspirin affects a rheumatic fever patient. We can do no better than turn to Dr. Paul Dudley White who while stating "that aspirin is the standard treatment in rheumatic fever," nevertheless pointed out that because "the possibility of long continued salicylate (aspirin) therapy may depress the production rate of immune bodies in the organism, it makes one hesitate to recommend such chronic treatment unreservedly."

"It is of considerable importance to recognize that evidence of the persistent activity of the rheumatic infection may be masked by the long continued use of salicylates which abolishes temporary symptoms and signs including fever and leucocytosis," Dr. White continued.[1]

In other words, long continued use of aspirin suppresses or masks the rheumatic infection, and actually interferes with the immunizing powers of the body. It should not take much to see how this can permanently damage the affected parts of the body.

Looking further, we find the *Journal of the American*

[1] Paul Dudley White, *Heart Disease.*

Medical Association, October 23, 1948, quoting Graham and Parker to the following effect:

"Sodium salicylate (a salt of aspirin) is widely used in the treatment of acute rheumatic fever and the more chronic forms of rheumatism. While there may be disagreements as to its precise value in the therapy of various rheumatic conditions there is general agreement that it is a toxic substance giving rise to a variety of untoward and even alarming symptoms which may interfere with its administration."[2]

The United States Dispensatory (20th Edition) states the following about aspirin:

"Overdoses of acetylsalicylic acid (aspirin) commonly produces ringing in the ears as do the inorganic salicylates. Frequently, however, even in quantities not excessive, it produces a very different type of intoxication. Among the most common symptoms are profuse sweating, cold extremities, either with or without a fall in body temperature, rapid or irregular pulse and occasionally albuminuria (albumin in the urine).

"In many reported cases there has been marked facial edema involving not only the skin but the mucous membrane of the mouth and throat."

Sidney O. Krassnoff and Mitchell Bernstein[3] pointed out that they "were able to find reports of only seven fatalities due to the acetylsalicylic acid (aspirin) in the American literature," but that "poisoning by this drug appears to be commoner in Europe, especially England," and then stated "that acetylsalicylic acid poisoning may be overlooked because of its mimicry of other toxic states."

"It is evident from the pathologic findings in our case, as well as in the fatal cases with necropsy (autopsy) reported by others that many of the symptoms and signs of acetylsalicylic acid (aspirin) poisoning are the result of changes chiefly in the brain, kidneys, and liver. The cerebral changes may result in a chain of symptoms varying from headache, dizziness, vertigo and tinnitus, down to stupor, coma and death," Krasnoff and Bernstein

---

[2] *Quarterly Journal of Medicine,* April 1948.

[3] "Acetylsalicylic Acid Poisoning," *Journal of the American Medical Association,* November 15, 1947.

pointed out, and then added that diseases of the central nervous system, psychosis, kidney diseases, the diseases of the liver, a simulation of diabetic coma due to metabolic changes from acidosis, may actually result from acetylsalicylic acid (aspirin) poisoning.

"Space does not permit a full consideration of the pharmacologic, toxicologic, and pathologic effects of 'aspirin' in relation to its manner of absorption, distribution in the body, excretion, toxic effects on the central nervous system, cardio-respiratory system and gastro-intestinal system, and hepatic, renal, and dermatologic manifestations," the authors stated. They then mentioned that "Hartman and others have pointed out that there appears to be no close relationship between the dosage of the salicylates and the toxic symptoms." They described two cases, one a 54-year-old man, the other a 5-month-old boy, in therapeutic doses of this drug proved fatal.

Cortisone and ACTH in Rheumatic Fever

In addition to aspirin, other drugs have been used in the treatment of rheumatic fever. Cortisone and ACTH are the drugs which have been tried most recently. Results of a three year study, undertaken by the American, British, and Canadian Heart Association "to determine whether ACTH, cortisone or aspirin is most effective in alleviating the symptoms of rheumatic fever," while so far inconclusive has, nevertheless, demonstrated "that there is little difference in the efficacy" of these remedies and that the dangers of side reaction with aspirin are much less.[4]

In discussing the relative merits of these remedies, a well-known physician pointed out that cortisone and ACTH are in reality more dangerous than aspirin because they are much more potent and have to be much more closely watched for side reactions affecting the pituitary, the adrenal, the thyroid, the pancreas, the kidneys, as well as the psyche (mind).

Now if these drugs are not the treatments of choice, what is the ideal treatment in these cases?

[4] *New York Times*, April 11, 1953.

Before answering this question, it might be well to see whether we could not at first determine how this disease develops.

If you should ask your doctor what causes rheumatic fever, he will, in all sincerity, tell you that he doesn't know, and that while a germ has been suspected, this is a mere guess. Here is how Levine puts it: "The exact etiology (cause) of this disease is not known although a streptococcus is thought by many to be the cause. The evidence, however, is very conflicting and the question is best regarded for the present as unanswered."[5]

Boyd states:

"It is always a matter of difficulty to demonstrate organisms in the lesions; when present, they are never numerous, and the fluid from the infected joints is nearly always sterile."[6]

MacCallum[7] explains it as follows:

"Although for years many investigators have attempted to show that it is caused by one sort of bacteria or other, generally some type of streptococcus—there is no convincing evidence that any of the different bacteria occasionally found in the blood or respiratory passages have any importance as its cause."

We can see from all this that the question of a germ being the cause is mere conjecture. Now, if the disease cannot be blamed on a germ, how does it develop? The answer is not so mysterious as it seems. Medical literature states that many predisposing factors play a role in its development.

"An important factor in the occurrence of the rheumatic infection and of rheumatic heart disease appears to be the social and economic status of the individual. These diseases are much more common, by several times at least, among the crowded poor than among the well-to-do inhabitants of almost every community. In the large American private schools, rheumatic fever, chorea, and rheumatic heart disease are uncommon, while in the large public schools they are relatively very common.

"Crowding, exposure to cold and wet without sufficient

---

[5] Dr. Samuel Levine, *Clinical Heart Disease.*

[6] Boyd, *Pathology of Internal Diseases.*

[7] MacCallum, *A Textbook of Pathology.*

protection, malnutrition and fatigue are probably all factors in producing this contrast," stated Paul Dudley White.[8]

Dealing with the same subject, Dr. Norman L. Moore[9] of the School of Nutrition, Cornell University, referred to observations conducted by Taran in 1941 which proved that the incidence of rheumatic recurrence was four times as high in the poor environment as in the good one.

"It has long been suggested that economic, sociologic, and dietary factors are concerned in some way in the etiology and recurrence of the disease. The above study gives emphasis to that point."

Here then, in clear and unequivocal terms, is an indication of why rheumatic fever develops. Malnutrition or poor dietary factors, fatigue, poor environment, or any of the influences which lower the resistance of the body, play an important role in the development of this disease.

The reason we have a preponderance of rheumatic fever among the poor is simply because the unfavorable factors mentioned above predominate in the homes of the poor.

However, since unfavorable influences are not limited exclusively to the poor, and since the children in well-to-do homes too, are often improperly nourished and exposed to influences which lead to over-fatigue, they are not altogether immune to it.

Improper food, excessive indulgence in sweets, the use of rich concentrated foods or refined foods, overeating, exhaustion, excessive emotional influences, are some of the many factors which affect the children of all classes.

White and Moore mentioned malnutrition and dietary factors as playing contributory roles. They did not mean lack of nutrition, but poor or inadequate nutrition.

Dr. Moore made this point clear when he stated that studies by Coburn and Moore in 1943, have given "positive evidence of the relationship between adequacy of diet and the susceptibility of the host of rheumatic fever" and continued further by specifying that "one of three factors in the genesis of the rheumatic state is conditioning of the host by a poor diet."

---

[8] Paul Dudley White, M.D., *Heart Disease.*

[9] "A New Approach to The Rheumatic Fever Problem," *New York State Journal of Medicine,* Jan. 1, 1949.

Dr. Moore further referred to the contribution by Jackson, Kelly, Rohret, and Duane 1947, who have proven that "the degree of deficiency of the diet was related to the incidence and degree of heart damage" and that "an excellent diet plus wholesome living conditions will practically eliminate the chances of recurrence with carditis (inflammation of the heart)."

Dr. Moore concluded by pointing out that observations have conclusively demonstrated that an incomplete or deficient diet plays an important role in the development of this disease and that a well-balanced diet plus wholesome living conditions will not only help toward rapid recovery but will protect the heart against damage.

The Best Treatment of Rheumatic Fever

Through all these facts, it should not be difficult to conclude what the most logical approach in these cases should be. Certainly not the use of suppressants, but the type of care which helps overcome the inflammatory process and aids in rebuilding the debilitated body. Rest, warmth, the use of hot baths, and the application of moist heat packs to the affected joints, plus good nursing and a carefully regulated nutritional program, make up an ideal approach in these cases.

How effective such a program is can be seen from the following case histories.

Ira was 8 years old when he became sick with rheumatic fever. The onset was sudden with high fever and excruciating pains and swelling in his legs and wrists.

The family physician who was called in and the specialist who joined him in consultation suggested the conventional treatment—aspirin at regular intervals, complete rest in bed, the application of heat to the inflamed joints, and what is usually considered "good, nourishing food." The physician was to see him daily to watch his progress and check his heart.

We need not describe the fear with which the parents received the information that their child was suffering from rheumatic fever. Most people know the dangers associated with this disease, and are terribly frightened by it. This may have been the reason for Ira's parents' refusal to go along with the conventional treatments and for their turning to our type of care.

Now followed an interesting period which was closely watched by family and friends. To the parents these were fearful days, while the other members of the family doubtfully shook their heads. Some even berated the parents for rejecting the standard type of treatment predicting that no good could come from it.

The treatments employed were simple. At first, plain lukewarm cleansing enemas, followed by hot epsom salt baths, were given twice daily. Following the bath, the boy was wrapped in sheets and rolled in blankets to induce perspiration.

The food during the first few days was limited to freshly squeezed orange and grapefruit juice, as well as other fruit juices.

For local relief, hot moist compresses were applied to the swollen and painful joints. Tepid spongings every two hours, to make the boy more comfortable, completed the routine.

Noticeable improvement became apparent within a few days. The temperature began to drop about the second or third day, and the swellings began to diminish materially. The pain lessened and sleep became more relaxed, less fitful.

After the first few days, the enemas and baths were reduced to one daily, and more substantial food was gradually introduced.

We began with small amounts of raw fruit. Then small meals of raw and steamed vegetables and raw and stewed fruit were gradually introduced to which a baked potato was added a few days later.

Each day brought further improvement, and after about three or four weeks, the boy was completely well.

During this time, no medication of any sort was used. It is interesting to mention at this point that the doctor who had first examined the boy and who was a close friend of the family watched the boy's progress closely, even though he was not officially in charge of the case. He knew that no medication was used, and while at first he had predicted all kinds of dire consequences, he ultimately was amazed to note how rapidly the boy recovered.

Neither he nor the specialist who reexamined the boy after he had completely recovered could discover any signs of heart disease.

Years later when Ira was inducted into the army cadet flying corps, a rigid checkup only confirmed that he was in excellent health.

The Story of Lydia C.

Here is another illustration of the effectiveness of this type of treatment:

Lydia C., four years old, came down with rheumatic fever. In checking over the child's history, we found that she had been suffering from asthma and other allergic conditions since birth, and that only a short time previous to her rheumatic attack had been subjected to a series of injections for these conditions.

Lydia was not suffering from painful joints but the examination left no doubt in the mind of the doctors that Lydia was suffering from a severe case of rheumatic fever.

The treatments in this case were practically a repetition of the other, with some minor modifications. Eliminative treatments and hydrotherapy (water applications) were used. Natural mineral and vitamin rich fruit juices were used during the first two or three days after which small meals of raw and stewed fruit, raw and steamed vegetables, and baked or steamed potatoes were introduced.

All other foods were at first completely excluded but the dairy products and small portions of chicken and lean meat were later permitted as the child improved.

It took over three weeks before the fever and heart symptoms were under complete control, and altogether about three months before the child had fully recovered. A cardiologist (heart specialist) called in to recheck the patient found everything in excellent condition!

It is interesting to note that not only did the patient recover from her rheumatic fever, but also that all former signs and symptoms of her allergic condition completely disappeared.

138

The patient is now a grown-up girl and in excellent health.

"You will never realize how frightened we were when the doctors told us how seriously ill Lydia was, and we will never forget what this rational regimen has done for her," her father stated only recently.

A report from the father of a boy who was afflicted with rheumatic fever should be of interest:

"In the winter of 1950-51, my son, Robert, aged 9, took ill. He felt weak, dispirited and tired. His bones ached and he had difficulty straightening out his body. This condition became more pronounced as the days passed despite constant regular attention. He was checked completely at a hospital to ascertain the nature of his illness, and spent a week there taking injections around the clock. A specialist decided that it was rheumatic fever and that Robert was to spend at least six months in bed. He was not to exert himself at all, and we were even to carry him to the bathroom. The boy's condition was gradually deteriorating, and in despair we turned to a doctor who employed hygienic, reconstructive therapies. Results were astonishing. Within one week he was able to straighten his body without effort. Two weeks later he was out of the house, and four weeks later he was playing ball with the other children, as if nothing ever happened. Needless to say, we owe this benefactor a great debt of gratitude."

These are only a few of many cases of rheumatic fever which have been treated with these simple rational measures, which have proven how easily such cases can be brought under control. In a practice extending over a period of fifty years, we have had occasion to observe many cases of rheumatic fever and in none of the cases which were treated by these conservative reconstructive methods from their inception, could any evidence of heart disease be detected as an aftermath of the acute condition.

The reason these methods are so successful is because they permit effective elimination of the deleterious substances by enabling the kidneys, the skin, as well as all other organs of elimination to function efficiently, give the body a chance to organize its own defenses, and bring about a reversal of the disease processes as rapidly as possible. Nothing is done to interfere with or suppress the body's restorative efforts.

The Dramatic Recovery of Lucy C.

In cases where the heart is already damaged, the problem is, of course, more difficult. However, even in such cases a discontinuance of the suppressive treatments and a change to the hygienic regimen often produces dramatic results.

Lucy C., ten years old, is a case in point. Lucy had a history of frequent colds and recurrent attacks of tonsilitis.

Her tonsils were finally removed but soon after, rheumatic fever developed. For months conventional treatments were employed, but Lucy only continued to grow worse.

On several occasions, friends tried to induce Lucy's parents to discontinue the conventional treatments and turn to the hygienic methods, but because of the dangers associated with this disease and the seriousness of Lucy's condition, they were afraid to try anything new. However, when the doctor in charge of the case mentioned that Lucy was "very low" and that he was surprised that she hadn't died "24 hours ago," the parents finally realized that they had nothing to lose and decided to make the change.

By that time, Lucy's heart was already badly damaged and greatly enlarged. Cor bovinum (ox heart) doctors call this type of heart. What was even more serious was that in addition to the enlarged and badly damaged heart, she was also suffering from a severe congestion of the lungs and showed all the signs of impending circulatory failure.

An examination by the physician revealed a low grade fever and a rapid pulse which was barely perceptible. Respiration was 46 per minute. No wonder the new physician too regarded the case as critical and couldn't hold out much hope!

Eliminative treatments were immediately instituted. All medication was discontinued. Warm cleansing enemas, mild hydrotherapy in the form of packs and hot foot baths, and a bland, vitamin and mineral rich diet was prescribed, which was later supplemented by meals which provided all essential nutritional needs of the body in easily digestible form.

It took about three weeks before we felt that we were on safe ground in this case. It is worth noting that at first Lucy's temperature began to rise, reaching as high as 103½, while her pulse slowed down and became much stronger, and her respiration grew much deeper and more regular.

The first ten days were days of extreme uncertainty, but after that we began to feel more confident. Another ten days or so, and the temperature, pulse and respiration were normal. From then on it was just a matter of continued rest in bed, adequate nutrition and good nursing care.

It took altogether about three to four months before Lucy had completely recovered and before she was permitted to leave her bed.

The last few weeks were rather difficult, for with the return of her health and strength, came the desire to get out of bed, and we had considerable difficulty to keep her at rest until we were sure that it was safe enough to permit her to get up.

Her happy mother explained Lucy's temperament by saying that she had always been a "tomboy" and that when well could outfight any boy her age in the block.

Lucy was seen again about 19 years later. She was then 29 years old, married, and the mother of a child.

While the defects of the heart could not be completely erased, the heart had become considerably smaller than it was at the time of her illness and had grown sufficiently strong to enable her to lead a normal life.

How Another Youngster Was Helped

The story of L. E. also illustrates what a sound physiological approach can accomplish, even in cases where permanent heart damage had already set in.

L. E. was 12 years old when she was stricken with rheumatic fever. For three months she was receiving conventional treatments, and by the time this new care was started, her heart was already badly affected. She was still running a temperature of about 103-104 and her joints were badly swollen and extremely tender and painful.

The suppressive remedies were promptly discontinued, and supportive and eliminative treatments in the form of enemas, hot foot baths and local compresses, applied to the painful joints, were started. In addition, a change from the deficient diet to a more suitable nutritional feeding program was initiated.

Before long, the temperature began to drop and the pains and swelling in the joints began to subside. Altogether the treatment continued for about three to four months. By that time, all pain and swelling had completely disappeared, her heart and circulation were fully compensated and Lucy was gradually able to resume her normal activities.

In view of the dangers inherent in rheumatic fever and the uncertain results associated with the conventional treatment, every parent should seriously consider this simple, physiological approach with its great restorative potentialities.

The Question of Allergy in Rheumatic Fever

In discussing the factors which predispose the body to acute rheumatic fever, the question of allergy is often brought up. Some maintain that acute rheumatic fever is an allergic disease and arises from the intake of foods or exposure to substances to which the body has become oversensitive.

The *Journal of the American Medical Association,* July 17, 1948,[10] editorially commented on the work done by Vaubel and Kling, later substantiated by Hall and Anderson, Rich and Gregory, as well as by Moore and Associates at the University of Southern California, which proved "That rheumatic fever is a reaction to parenteral contact with foreign protein to which tissues previously had been sensitized" and that the human rheumatic heart, by the same token, also arises from "parenteral contact with foreign protein to which the cardiac tissues have been previously sensitized."

---

[10] "Allergic Carditis."

In other words, rheumatic fever affecting the heart, as well as the other organs and parts of the body, arises from an allergy to a foreign protein, which, getting into the body by ways other than the digestive system, irritates the tissues or parts of the body which have become sensitive to it.

The first question that naturally arises in connection with this is what causes an allergic condition? If we re-read the reports of Heiser, Pottenger, et al., we will find that incorrect nutrition plays a vital role in the development of allergy.

Another question then follows: Assuming the body has become sensitized (allergic), what are these foreign proteins which set the vicious cycle in motion? To obtain the answer to this, it is well to bear in mind that the superfluous vaccines and serums are foreign proteins. In the light of the above, isn't it possible that Lydia's attack of rheumatic fever, following the multiple injections in the treatment of her "allergic" conditions actually contributed to the onset of this disease?

While the editorial quoted above tries to make a case for the streptococcus, since the streptococcus too is a foreign protein, we wonder whether a much stronger case could not be made against the use of vaccines and serums which are much more dangerous than is generally recognized.

Incidentally, Homer F. Swift (*Medicine*, September 1940) from the Hospital of the Rockefeller Institute for Medical Research, who, while mentioning that "the disease has all the earmarks of being infectional in nature" and that "at present, a hemolytic (blood destroying) streptococcus seems to bear a more intimate relationship to the disease than any other known pathogenic agent," nevertheless stated that "it is now generally admitted that multiple causative factors are operative in the pathogenesis of many diseases; and particularly does this seem to be true in rheumatic fever and rheumatic heart disease."[11]

Currier McEwen from the Hospital of the Rockefeller Institute for Medical Research, Dean of New York and Bellevue Hospital Medical College, quoted Glover, who stated that "no disease has a clearer cut social incidence

[11] *Medicine*, September 1940.

than acute rheumatism which falls perhaps thirty times as frequently upon the poorer children of the industrial town as upon the children of the well-to-do," and then pointed out that the British Medical Research Council indicated that "the high incidence among the poor is probably due to the malnutrition, dirt, crowding and other bad hygienic conditions following in the wake of poverty."[12]

Rheumatic Heart Disease

The type of heart disease which manifests itself as an aftermath of rheumatic fever is known as valvular heart disease and/or endocarditis.

In this type of heart disease, the damage affects primarily the valves of the heart. Scars form on and around the valves of the heart and this prevents them from closing or opening completely. If you remember, the valves of the heart open to empty the blood from the upper chamber into the lower chamber and then close to prevent the blood from flowing back. When the valves are damaged, they are unable to close or open completely and as a result, the blood either fails to flow through entirely or some of it is forced back. This places a great strain on the heart and forces it to enlarge.

Our Power to Rebuild Health

Health can be rebuilt only when we work with and not against the healing powers of the body. Our body is constantly trying to ward off influences inimical to health, but we often misinterpret these efforts and interfere with what the body is trying to accomplish. A rise or fall in blood pressure, the changes in the heart beat, an increase in the number of white blood cells, a rise in temperature, a running nose, a cough, skin eruptions, vomiting spells, diarrhea, are all efforts on the part of the body to rid itself of inimical substances and overcome or counteract conditions which endanger life.

[12] *Hospital Social Service,* Supplement 2.

While these acute reactions are unpleasant and often painful, they nevertheless play a very important role in the restoration of health and the preservation of life. Suppressive treatments in any form interfere with these health restoring efforts on the part of the body and ultimately lead to an exhaustion of the body's protective functions, often causing irreparable damage, even though they temporarily camouflage or mask the symptoms of the disease and provide a measure of relief.

CHAPTER XIV

THE ERA OF THE GREAT DELUSION

"The Young Physician starts life with twenty drugs for each disease and the old physician ends life with one drug for twenty diseases." Dr. William Osler.

In this chapter, we are going to deal with a subject which can be highly explosive and lead to a great deal of confusion, unless properly understood. We are alluding to the almost universal reliance on drugs in the treatment of disease.

It seems to us that we are living in the era of the great delusion. Life is filled with delusions, which upon closer examination are found to be wanting. One of the greatest of our present day delusions, however, is the popular belief that drugs can cure our ills.

The reverse is actually true. Not only do drugs fail to rebuild health, they often cause a vast amount of harm.

Let us turn to medical literature and see whether this is not the case. *The U. S. Dispensatory* (the most authoritative book on drugs) writes the following about quinine, one of the drugs in common use:

"Even in the quantities employed for therapeutic purposes quinine frequently produces unpleasant symptoms. The most common of these is ringing in the ears often accompanied with a sensation of fullness in the head, and perhaps some obtunding (blunting) of the sense of hearing."

With the use of larger doses, these symptoms become intensified:

"The deafness is very marked, disturbed vision may exist, and the flushed face, with the sense of distension in the head, may point towards a cerebral congestion which is in some cases relieved by spontaneous epistaxis (nose bleed)."

Another drug often used in the treatment of disease is iodine. Most of us know that iodine is applied externally as a disinfectant, but how many are aware that it is also prescribed for internal use? Here is what the *Dispensatory* states about this drug, when taken internally:

"Even in medicinal doses it sometimes causes alarming symptoms, such as fever, restlessness, disturbed sleep, palpitations, excessive thirst, acute pain in the stomach, vomiting and purging, violent cramps, frequent pulse, and finally, progressive emaciation if the medicine is not laid aside."

Incidentally, even when applied externally, iodine can be harmful since it can be absorbed through the skin.

The bromides are another class of drugs which produce unpleasant and toxic symptoms. Dr. Lewis P. Gundry in the *JAMA* stated that headache, anorexia, dizziness, tremors, fatigue, irritability, poor memory and transitory mental confusion are some of the early symptoms of bromide intoxication, and that if the medication is continued, or the dose increased, the symptoms of mild intoxication, restlessness, weakness, thick speech and unsteady gait become clinical features.[1]

One of the insidious dangers in drug medication is their tendency to accumulate in the system. Though not always immediately apparent, detrimental effects can show up most unexpectedly, and be quite severe or even cause death.

Here is what the *U. S. Dispensatory* says about the cumulative effect of bromides:

"As the drug is eliminated very slowly, when used continuously, it tends to accumulate in the system and in sufficient doses may give rise to the phenomena known as bromism. The symptoms are muscular weakness, general mental and bodily sluggishness, loss of memory, often marked sleepiness, depression of spirits deepening into complete apathy, lowering of temperature, and finally scarcely more than a feeble automation." And further:

"Despite the fact that it leaves the system through practically all the excretory organs, having been found in

[1] "Bromide Intoxication," August 5, 1939.

the sweat, saliva, urine, and intestinal mucus, it is eliminated very slowly and has been found in the urine as much as a month after the last dose . . . "

Dr. Theodore Cornbleet, University of Illinois Dermatologist, in a talk at the ninety-ninth annual meeting of the American Medical Association, pointed out that "the drug (bromides) which piles up in the body because of the system's inability to pass it off readily, will in some persons bring on simulated psychoses, such as manic depression, which persists until the drug is counteracted," and then stated, "that perhaps as much as 5 percent of the nation's mental illness could be attributed to misuse of the drug."[2]

Wohl and Robertson emphasized that chronic bromide intoxication is not an uncommon occurrence and then went on to state that "symptoms of bromism may mimic almost any neuropsychiatric state and are frequently blurred by an underlying condition for which bromides are given."[3]

The Untimely Death of Robert Walker

The untimely death of Robert Walker, well known motion picture actor, is only one case history which illustrates the dangers of drugs which accumulate in the system.

It was reported that Robert Walker collapsed following the taking of a dose of sodium amytal. According to the press, he had been using this drug for some time on the advice of his doctor without any apparent ill effects, and that on the evening previous to his collapse took his usual dose of medicine. His collapse followed and was diagnosed as the result of "circulation failure."

When death follows from the use of any of these drugs, it is caused because the functioning of the heart, the breathing, or the circulation has stopped. This is then diagnosed as death due to "cardiac standstill," "respiratory failure," or "circulatory collapse."

Dr. Victor Cefalu, Assistant County Coroner, pointed

---

2 *New York Herald Tribune*, July 1, 1950.

3 "Bromide Intoxication," *Transactions of American Therapeutic Society*, 1941.

out that sodium amytal has a cumulative effect, and did not mince any words in telling us that he regarded this as the reason for the "circulatory failure" in Robert Walker's case.

It is well to bear in mind that the harmful effects of drugs may continue unrecognized for a long time, and then show up most unexpectedly.

In our *New Hope for Arthritis Sufferers,* we quoted Dr. Irving S. Cutter, Dean of the Medical School, Northwestern University, Chicago, who in his discussion of chincophen, a drug employed in the treatment of gout, mentioned that this drug is extremely harmful and therefore must be carefully watched:

"Unfortunately, the toxic effects may come on suddenly with so much injury to vital structures that nothing can be done to save life," Dr. Cutter stated.

It is needless to stress the fact that the harmful effects of the drugs are often not recognized because they simulate or mimic other diseases.

The Antibiotics

Among the remedies most recently introduced are the antibiotics or the so-called "miracle" or "wonder" drugs, such as penicillin, streptomycin, aureomycin and chloromycetin.

These "miracle" or "wonder" drugs are regarded as the last word in medicine and are considered most effective in the treatment of our so-called "infectious" diseases. The fact is, however, that these drugs are effective merely as suppressants and not as cures.

At a recent conference held under the auspices of the New York Academy of Sciences, Biology Section, many of the authorities present explained that the antibiotics "merely hold the infection in check as long as significantly high levels of antibiotics are actually present in the blood stream" and that "when the antibiotics are discontinued, a patient may suffer a relapse."[4]

A fact which is now gradually emerging is that while the antibiotics are suppressing the symptoms of disease,

[4] *New York Times,* January 18, 1952.

they also, in the words of Dr. Abraham S. Gordon, "undermine the system by which the human body produces disease killing antibodies."[5]

This incidentally is true of all drugs which act as suppressants.

Another fact now gradually being recognized is that these drugs are not selective in the type of bacteria they hold in check and while suppressing or checking the action of the disease bacteria, they also undermine or destroy the function of essential bacteria in the digestive organs, often causing serious intestinal and ano-rectal diseases.

Dr. Sylvan D. Manhem in an article in the *New York State Journal of Medicine* pointed out "that the administration of these drugs resulted in ano-rectal complications which in some instances were severe enough to require surgical treatment" and that these "complications apparently result because the normal intestinal flora is destroyed."[6]

In an article in the *U. S. Armed Forces Medical Journal*, Captain Robert L. Gilman[7] called penicillin an allergic hazard and reported "that reactions in presensitized patients are marked by chills, fever, prostration, arthritis symptoms, and shock" and then continued to point out that recovery from these reactions "takes a long time and there may be serious relapse."

Dr. Alton Ochsner,[8] Chairman of the Department of Surgery of the Tulane University School of Medicine, in a report delivered at the thirteenth Congress of the International Society of Surgery referred to the dangers of the antibiotics in surgery, and pointed out that a marked increase in deaths from thrombo-embolism (the formation of clots in the veins) has taken place from the use of these drugs in surgery.

Out of 580 cases of thrombo-embolism at Charity Hospital in New Orleans, 203 cases ended in death from pulmonary embolism, a condition in which the clot reaches the lung, Dr. Ochsner mentioned, and then went on to

5 *New York Times*, May 11, 1955.
6 *New York Times*, January 6, 1952.
7 *Time*, October 30, 1950.
8 "Anti-biotic Peril Seen By Surgeon," *New York Times*, Oct. 13, 1949.

say that "the increased incidence of thrombo-embolism and the increased number of fatal cases from pulmonary embolism is probably due to the increased coagulability of the blood resulting from the almost routine administration of antibiotics to all hospital patients."

That the antibiotics can cause death is apparent from many medical reports. Dr. Abraham Rosenthal, Assistant Medical Examiner in Brooklyn, reported that eight people were killed by penicillin in Brooklyn in the last two years and "that the eight—none seriously ill—died within minutes after injection from massive allergic reactions."[9]

The dangers of chloromycetin, one of the more recent antibiotics, and the fatalities that resulted from its use are now history. The *Journal of the American Medical Association* in a series of articles, July 5 and August 2, 1952, called attention to the dangers of this drug, while *Time Magazine* reported that a quick and thorough check by top-notch authorities found that "chloromycetin was connected with the deaths of at least 72 aplastic anemia victims."[10]

Ethan Allan Brown[11] of Boston, dealing with this point as it relates to the antibiotics, referred to "today's enthusiastic but haphazard use of antibiotics as 'appalling' " and then went on to say:

"It is misleading to speak only of patients whose deaths are recorded as resulting from reactions to anti-biotics," since "there are more deaths which do not get into print."

"Still more numerous are serious reactions short of death. Finally there are countless allergic reactions," he continued.

"In many cases, allergic reactions are not reported because the patient did not die from them. What the medical reports fail to stress is how many had wished themselves dead." Dr. Brown further asserted that he was one of those exquisitely sensitive to penicillin who wished himself dead.

Dealing specifically with the subject of penicillin, Drs. Samuel M. and Alan R. Feinberg, in a guest editorial in the *Journal of the American Medical Association*,[12]

9 *New York Post*, May 17, 1954.
10 *Time*, August 25, 1952.
11 *Time*, November 9, 1953.
12 "Allergy to Penicillin," *JAMA*, March 3, 1956.

pointed out that the incidence of allergic reactions "in different groups varies from 1 to 5%" and that many fatalities resulted from this medication. "We know personally of a number of fatal cases that have not been reported," the authors stated.

"There are a variety of types of allergic reaction to penicillin," the authors mentioned and then went on to say: "cutaneous (skin) manifestations include urticaria, rashes, exfoliative dermatitis, contact dermatitis, and erythema nodosum and multiforme. Purpura has been noted. Increasing numbers of instances of periarteritis are reported."

"The serum-sickness syndrome consists of urticaria and arthralgria and swelling of joints, frequently fever and albuminuria, and sometimes visceral[13] and nervous system changes," the authors continued.

Of additional interest to us is their mentioning that "a number of papers describe myocardial (heart) and renal (kidney) changes occurring during the serum sickness type of reaction."

The harmful results occurred whether the medication was administered in the form of an injection, taken by mouth, inhaled, taken in the form of a lozenge, or applied externally to the skin, the authors pointed out.

That most drugs are poisonous is well known. What is not so well known is that drugs are poisonous even when taken in small or medicinal doses. Thienes and Haley *(Clinical Toxicology)* classify the drugs used in ordinary medical practice such as aspirin, quinine, the barbiturates [phenobarbital, sodium amytal] bromide, atrophine, codeine, belladonna, caffeine, aconite, cinchophen, morphine, mercury, arsenic, the sulfa drugs, the hormones like thyroid, and such drugs as digitalis (which is classed as cardiac poison), as well as the nitrites (nitroglycerin and amyl-nitrite) dicoumarol and heparin (which are used in different types of heart disease to counteract clotting), under such headings as convulsant poisons, central nervous system poisons, poisons acting on nerve trunks, ganglia and nerve endings, muscle poisons, protoplasmic (tissue)

---

[13] Dictionary definition of viscera—the internal organs, especially those of the cavities of the body, as the heart, liver, intestines, etc.

poisons and poisons of the blood and hematopiotic (blood-making) organs.

Marion B. Sulzberger and Victor H. Witten[14] in *Postgraduate Medicine* mentioned that "fatal reactions to drugs are not altogether uncommon," and then pointed out that "not only dermatologists, but also physicians in general are now recognizing the ever increasing incidence of dermatoses (skin diseases) due to drugs.

"In addition to the skin, other organs and systems also may be affected; for example, blood changes, fever, delirium and shock may be present," Sulzberger and Witten continued.

The Effects of Drugs on the Heart and the Circulatory System

According to Thienes and Haley, such drugs as the barbiturates, arsenic, the coal tar analgetics, digitalis, insulin, mercury, nitrites, quinidine and quinine, may cause circulatory collapse; digitalis, ephedrine, quinine and quinidine may cause brachycardia or a slowing of the pulse; atropine, benzedrine, ephedrine, epinephrine, nitrites, and thyroid, may cause tachycardia or a rapid pulse beat; aconite, digitalis, epinephrine, ephedrine and thyroid may cause heart irregularities; ephedrine and epinephrine may cause hypertension or high blood pressure; aconite, arsenic, barbiturates, coal tar analgetics, and nitrites may cause low blood pressure; ephedrine, epinephrine, lead and nicotine may cause constriction or spasms in the blood vessels; arsenic, dicoumarol, heparin, sulfonamides, and thiouracil, may cause hemorrhage; while arsenic, barbital, lead, morphine, sulfonamides, nitrites, and thiouracil, may cause various disorders of the blood.

Isn't it logical to conclude that any remedy or drug which can interfere with the function of the heart and circulation can ultimately cause permanent damage? This is the reason the progressive physician recognizes the importance of working with the forces of the body and places his reliance on sound physiological principles, rather than on remedies which merely camouflage the symptoms of disease, and thereby distort the picture.

[14] "Allergic Dermatoses Due to Drugs," June, 1952.

While the number of dead reported from medication may not seem large when the vast number of people who submit to it is considered, if the number of dead which are not reported as having been caused by the drugs or which go unrecognized, and the countless people who become affected by them short of death and who become either temporarily or permanently disabled are taken into consideration, then the picture is indeed formidable.

The Physiological Approach to Health Restoration

If people cannot rely on drugs for help, what are they to do in case of illness? This is a logical question, and a point which must be clearly understood if we are to avoid the confusion which can easily engulf us. However, before this question can be answered, a clear picture of how disease develops and what the different symptoms which show up in disease signify, must be obtained.

The great mistake in the conventional treatment of disease is the failure to recognize the underlying causes of diseases, and because of this we are unable to understand what the symptoms which appear in disease mean. We then blame many of our diseases on germs and viruses and are content when an anti-biotic or any of the other drugs of a suppressive nature relieves the annoying or frightening symptoms of the disease. We overlook the fact that any measure or treatment which controls or subdues the symptoms of disease without eliminating the underlying causes, cannot restore health.

Furthermore, it is well to recognize the fact that while these remedies check or subdue the symptoms of disease, they also impair the body's ability to produce its own disease killing anti-bodies and this ultimately leads only to more extensive damage.

Dr. Abraham S. Gordon, Chief of the Arthritis Clinic, Kings County Hospital and Jewish Hospital in Brooklyn, in an address before the Medical Society of the State of New York, pointed this out very clearly.

"Antibiotics have been, and still are a great advance in anti-microbial therapeutics. The little animalculae (bacteria) have been caught by surprise and they are retreating before the onslaught of our new weapons," he stated, and then continued:

"But in the perspective of time this victory is only temporary. A battle has been won but the war is still on, and the enemy is quite formidable. Some day in the future, and we see some signs of it now, the bacteria will develop a resistance to all antibiotics and it is a question whether we can keep a step ahead of them forever."

He then went on to say that "recent medical evidence suggests that the wide use of antibiotics has altered benign bacteria into agents capable of causing disease; in other cases, new forms of disease appear," and then listed such diverse diseases as asthma, migraine, necrosis (degeneration of tissue), anemia, tuberculosis, rheumatic fever and skin ailments, among those which develop.

Dr. Gordon's clear-sighted approach to this important question should make us realize that our major need is to correct the underlying causes of disease and not to be content with mere palliation.

CHAPTER XV

THE ELUSIVE MICROORGANISMS

The changes which manifest themselves in disease develop in response to a need and result from an attempt on the part of the body to cope with a problem. This applies not only to the symptoms of disease such as fever, pain, inflammation, diarrhea, cough, skin eruptions, etc., but also to many of the physical or structural changes which take place in the tissues and organs of the body, as well as in the surrounding areas.

We have seen that the heart increases in size and that scars and thickening develop in the muscle walls and in and around the valves of the heart in response to a need; to make it possible for the heart to cope with a difficult or dangerous situation and to enable it to do its work.

Why not recognize that when germs or viruses multiply and become virulent that this too may be the outgrowth of a need and part of the body's defense mechanism?

Many scientists have come to realize that germs or viruses multiply and become virulent when the body is in an inferior state of health and that the antibiotics or other drugs while often able to suppress or inhibit the functions of the germs or viruses, fail to correct or remove the underlying disease condition. These scientists are aware that germs or viruses multiply and become more virulent in disease because the diseased condition provides a favorable soil for their growth and development, and that to check their growth and development, the diseased condition must be corrected or changed.

Germs and viruses are virulent or benign and multiply or are kept in check depending upon the medium in which they live. They become active and virulent when dead or foreign substances provide a favorable soil for their growth and development, and become inactive or benign when the dead or foreign material has been eliminated or the body's immunizing and self-protective powers have succeeded in establishing a state of tolerance or compensation.

That germs and viruses are not major causes of disease and thrive and become virulent only when the soil is favorable, can be seen from the fact that when transplanted from one medium or soil into another, their characteristics change in conformity with the medium in which they are transplanted. This demonstrates that the soil determines the type and the activity of the germ or virus, and proves further that the soil or its environment is the activating force.

This also explains why germs or viruses which at first are held at bay by the antibiotics or some other suppressive drugs ultimately develop a resistance to them, often causing the disease to recur with greater virulence or to erupt in a new and more severe form.

Dr. Rene J. Dubos of the Rockefeller Institute has made this point clear when in a talk before the National Institute of Health Scientists, he stated that there is strong evidence "that bacteria and viruses become dangerous only when the setup is right for them. Otherwise, even the most virulent of them is harmless," and then pointed out that "every person carries in the body throughout life a host of supposedly deadly 'microbes' which live in blood and tissues as harmless guests until something happens to send them on a rampage."

"Although the presence of the right microorganisms is necessary for the particular disease, the real cause of the 'something' or combination of 'something' is a matter of which the present day physician is usually quite ignorant," Dr. Dubos pointed out, and then went on to say that "there even is danger that doctors who eliminate one form of supposedly malignant microorganism with some extremely potent new drugs are just making room in the body for the increase of some worse kind."

Now what is this "something" or "combination of something" of which many of our present day physicians are quite ignorant?

Dr. Dubos answered this question at a conference of the American Foundation where he pointed out that "normally the microorganisms that are all around us are held in check" and that "a transient proliferation of the microorganism or disease" develops "when the resistance of the body is overcome by a toxic or traumatic experience."[1]

Dr. Maclyn McCarthy of the Rockefeller Institute for Medical Research is another one who recognized this fact. In discussing the relationship of the streptococcus to rheumatic fever, he pointed out that "only in certain individuals and only in certain circumstances did streptococcus lead directly to rheumatic fever," and then continued to say that "the secret of the mechanisms involved in the pathogenesis (causes) of the disease seems to reside in some sort of interaction between the streptococcus and the susceptible human host."[2]

How Disease Arises

At this point, a short discussion of the two types of disease, the acute and chronic disease, should be of interest.

An acute disease arises when the body's defensive mechanism attempts to eliminate or counteract toxins or other elements of a noxious nature which have been generated within the body or have been taken into the system with food and drink or in the form of chemicals or drugs.

We observe that in acute disease, many of our bodily functions become intensified or accelerated. Increased temperature, rapid pulse, quick shallow breathing, inflammation and pain are some of the symptoms which show that the body is engaged in an effort to fight off or rectify an abnormal condition.

Authorities are aware that these intensified functions arise because of a need and serve a constructive purpose. It should, therefore, be apparent that the use of any modality which suppresses these symptoms in reality interferes with the body's rectifying efforts and endangers life.

---

[1] "Research Need Cited by Experts," *New York Times,* Nov. 16, 1945.

[2] *New York Times,* November 30, 1955

Our task in acute disease is to help the body accomplish its task as quickly and as effectively as possible and not disrupt or interfere with these efforts. Drugs which suppress these symptoms not only frustrate these efforts of the body to correct the abnormal or unhealthy conditions but actually create more damage. This is the reason acute diseases recur in many instances, and often even in a more intensive form.

Chronic Disease

When the defensive or recuperative powers of the body are effectively broken down or suppressed, they are unable to overcome or counteract the noxious or harmful influences, and a chronic condition or a disease in which degenerative changes gain the upper hand, has its beginning.

Medicine recognizes this fact. Harold G. Wolff,[3] Professor of Medicine, Cornell University, Medical College, quoted Claude Bernard, who "saw 'disease' as an outcome of adaptation to noxious forces in which the responses, though appropriate, are faulty in amount" and then continued by stating that "in this concept, the individual is damaged through the wrong magnitude of adaptive responses whether too much or too little."

This is merely another way of saying that "disease" develops when the defensive mechanism of the body cannot overcome the noxious or unwholesome influences thoroughly or completely, and proves that the use of any remedy which masks or suppresses the symptoms of disease and thereby hampers the effective working of the defense mechanism of the body, actually contributes to the development of chronic and degenerative diseases.

We have indicated before that rectal and intestinal disorders often follow the use of the antibiotics. We have also seen that permanent heart damage often follows the use of suppressive drugs in rheumatic fever. It is also well known that many people are "not quite the same" after "recovering" from an acute disease. An impairment in hearing, disturbance in vision, nervousness, chronic fatigue,

---

[3] "Stress and Adaptive Patterns Resulting in Tissue Damage in Man," *The Medical Clinics,* May 1955.

rheumatic pains, etc., are some of the disturbances which show up after their apparent recovery.

In our *New Hope For Arthritis Sufferers,* we quoted W. G. MacCallum who stated the following, in connection with fever, one of the acute symptoms in disease:

"Only in the last decade has it become vaguely appreciated that there is real evidence that fever on the contrary, is a reaction elaborated to a considerable degree of perfection which aids in the defense of the body against the advance of an injurious agent by facilitating the production of the substances which are formed in the body to neutralize poisons or kill bacteria.

"From this point of view it would seem, to say the least, shortsighted to give a patient in fever an antipyretic (antifever) drug which will cut short the febrile (fever) reaction," Dr. MacCallum concluded.[4]

Selye referred to the findings of the Austrian psychiatrist, Wagner Jauregg, who recognized "the therapeutic action of fever in various mental diseases, especially general paralysis."

Dr. O. P. J. Falk,[5] Assistant Professor of Clinical Medicine, St. Louis University School of Medicine, compared the results obtained in acute respiratory infections such as colds and influenza when treated with the usual aspirin combinations and with milk sugar tablets, and pointed out that the "aspirin and phenacetin treated cases . . . had about twice the period of disability" than those treated with the milk sugar tablets, adding that the "physiologic disadvantages of aspirin and phenacetin" result from the fact "that fever is artificially reduced."

Dr. Falk also went on to say that "a considerable increase in the percentage of complications occurred in the aspirin treated group."

Drs. Vincent W. Archer, George Cooper, Jr. and Norman Adair, of the Department of Roentgenology, University of Virginia Hospital, in a report presented before the 96th Annual Convention of the American Medical Association, had this to say on the subject:

"It is the almost universal experience of physicians in the larger reference institutions that an increasing

---

[4] *A Textbook of Pathology.*
[5] "Aspirin and Anti-biotics," *Prevention,* December 1954.

number of patients are seen in whom the classical symptoms of disease are masked or modified by previous chemotherapy (drugs)" and then quoted among others Rothman, who "summarized the literature through 1945, stressing the recurrence of symptoms following cessation of chemotherapy."[6]

Fourteen cases in which penicillin and the sulpha-drugs, used separately or in combination, suppressed the initial conditions, only to recur in more serious or virulent form after the drugs were discontinued, were also described by these authors.

Regarding the effect of the antibiotics in surgical emergencies, the *Journal of the American Medical Association* quoted F. R. Cole who in the *American Journal of Surgery* stated that their use "may distort the symptoms as well as the objective findings" and that while "they reduce the fever and abdominal symptoms and normalize the leucocyte count . . . the pathological process continues, and thrombosis of vessels with gangrene and rupture may occur."[7]

It should not be difficult to understand why Dr. Abraham S. Gordon, Chief of The Arthritis Clinic at Kings County Hospital and Jewish Hospital in Brooklyn, N. Y., stated that following the use of antibiotics such diverse diseases as asthma, migraine, necrosis (tissue degeneration), anemia, tuberculosis, rheumatic fever, and skin ailments often develop.

How Should an Acute Disease Be Treated?

Now if these remedies do not really restore the health of the patient, in what way can it be regained?

At the outset, let us not forget that in acute disease the body's defense mechanism is working overtime to rid itself of, or neutralize, toxins or elements of a poisonous nature, and that the symptoms which manifest themselves during this stage are merely indications of this effort on the part of the organism.

[6] "Symptoms Masked or Modified by Chemotherapy," *JAMA,* October 30, 1948.
[7] "Masking of Acute Abdominal Conditions with Antibiotics," *JAMA,* June 7, 1952.

It should seem that the only logical course to follow during this period would be to provide the body with the care which will aid it in accomplishing its purpose.

That is what we are trying to do when we employ or suggest the natural means which are at our disposal. The measures we employ help to eliminate the toxins and aid in rebuilding the immunizing and recuperative forces of the body. We avoid all methods which suppress symptoms and retard or interfere with the body's recuperative processes.

We provide rest and quiet, make use of the simple warm water enema to cleanse the bowels, and apply packs, baths or other forms of hydrotherapy to promote better elimination. We restrict the intake of food, using only fluids or, at most, a minimum of the easily digestible foods. The emphasis is on plenty of rest, quiet, good nursing, and a minimum of food or abstinence from food until the acute condition is brought under control.

This type of care accelerates the elimination of toxins by way of the kidneys, the skin, as well as the other organs of elimination, and helps in restoring the body to health.

As an illustration of how this method works, the case of L. R. is of particular interest.

Mr. R. suffered from chest pains with recurrent attacks of fever which were accompanied by extreme loss of appetite and extreme debility.

During these attacks, his vision would become completely blurred, but would clear up as soon as the fever subsided.

When Mr. R. visited us for the first time, he brought along a copy of the diagnosis from his physician, who was also a personal friend. It read as follows:

"Diffuse vascular disease involving retinal vessels, coronary vessels and probably mesentary vessels of abdomen.

"Symptoms: Periodic episodes of fever, blurred vision, chest pains, gastro-intestinal disturbance."

Translated into simple language, this meant that his periodic episodes of fever, blurred vision, chest pains, and digestive disorders were caused by a disease of the blood vessels of the eyes, the heart, and the abdomen.

Sometime later, Mr. R. brought along a copy of a letter forwarded to his doctor by a well known specialist. After mentioning that an electro-cardiogram revealed evidence of coronary occlusion, the specialist went on to say, among other things:

"This patient presents a rather bizarre and complicated picture. The recurrent episodes of fever, for about two years . . . together with more recent episodes of gaseousness and anorexia (lack of appetite) at about two month intervals, for over two years, are unusual manifestations. The persistent elevation of the sedimentation rate may be important. The hemorrhages which you observed in the left eye ground with some exudate . . . is important. All of these symptoms suggest some diffuse process, probably a diffuse vascular disease or lupus."

These attacks recurred at regular intervals and when they occurred, the patient was treated with cortisone. It usually took about two weeks before the fever and the other symptoms subsided, but they kept on recurring about every two months.

The patient was discouraged and badly frightened.

At the outset we made it clear to him that we would take his case only on condition that when the next attack occurred, he would use no medication but would follow our instructions.

He agreed, and not long after, the typical attack with all its symptoms set in.

When this happened, his friend, the doctor, again advised cortisone, but the patient informed him that this time he would try to work out the problem without drugs.

It took about two weeks before the fever and the other symptoms subsided. While the patient was quite worried about it at first, the fact that the condition cleared up without the use of drugs had a most dramatic effect in raising his morale, and inspired him with new hope.

Following his recovery from this attack, the patient was warned not to slip back into his old routine of living but to continue with the regimen which we outlined for him.

No further recurrences have taken place and after a few months of this type of living, the patient was advised that he could again return to an active and normal life.

It is now more than fifteen years since the patient

started with this regimen, and during all this time has had no return of these attacks.

It is interesting to mention that about six months after following this regimen, our patient visited his physician friend who, after subjecting him to a most thorough examination, exclaimed, "I don't know what you have been doing, but whatever it is, keep it up! It has made a new man out of you!"

What To Do in Chronic Diseases

In chronic disease we have an entirely different picture. This type of disease develops when the body is unable to react effectively to the toxic accumulations in the system, and as a result gives rise to various degenerative changes.

Our aim in these cases is to reawaken the body's curative powers so that they may again react to the harmful accumulations and make the necessary efforts to restore the health of the body.

Stating it a little differently, we employ the kind of care which strengthens and rebuilds the body's recuperative powers so that they can begin to do an efficient job of cleansing and rebuilding. In other words, we try to convert a chronic disease back to an acute condition, for this is the condition in which the body is actively engaged in ridding itself of the offending influences and in restoring health.

A carefully regulated nutritional program, emotional control, plenty of rest and sleep, exercises adjusted to the individual need, plus the application of heat and other rational physiologic measures, carefully applied over a period of time in accordance with the need of the case, help to accomplish this purpose.

It is needless to say that the diseases of a chronic or degenerative nature are much more difficult to handle than the acute diseases and in most instances, take much longer to respond. Furthermore, it is well to bear in mind that the degenerative processes may have proceeded to a point where it may be impossible to correct the damage completely. However, this is the only approach which will accomplish all that is possible in the circumstances.

CHAPTER XVI

HOW ABOUT THE DRUGS USED IN HEART DISEASE?

At this point, the question naturally arises: What can be done for a person whose heart is already damaged, and are the drugs which are applied in these cases of any help?

We wish to reiterate what we have stated before, namely, that no drugs actually restore health, they merely modify or suppress the symptoms of disease. This holds true with equal force to the drugs which are used in heart disease. While it is true that in an emergency, one may feel that there is no alternative but to resort to these drugs, it is well to bear in mind that while these drugs may provide temporary relief, they can also cause a great deal of harm, and that because of this, a well regulated program of care along the lines outlined in this book offers the only sound approach.

The drugs most often used in heart disease are digitalis, the mercurial diuretics and the nitrites (amyl nitrate and nitroglycerine).

The Effect of Digitalis

A sick heart is a weak and damaged heart. The heart does not possess the strength to contract fully and as a result is unable to maintain a healthy circulation. In an effort to make up for its shortcomings, it is often forced to work much faster, pumping many more times per minute. This prevents it from getting enough rest between beats and in time causes it to become completely worn out.

165

Digitalis causes an increase in the contraction of the heart and slows down the number of heart beats per minute. This improves the circulation and provides the heart with greater intervals of rest.

It is needless to say that because digitalis affects the heart this way, it often provides dramatic relief. However, it is well to bear in mind that the relief is only of a temporary nature and that no permanent correction is possible unless the muscle of the heart is strengthened and rebuilt.

There is another aspect which must be considered in connection with digitalis. What are its permanent effects on the heart when used over a period of time?

An investigation will reveal that digitalis is a poison, and if not stopped in time, can cause a great deal of damage to the heart.

In an article, "Digitoxin Intoxication," Dr. Arthur M. Master quoted von Jacksch who in his book on poisons, stated:

"Digitalin and digitoxin (digitalis preparations) are frightful cardiac (heart) poisons. Their use at the bedside necessitates the greatest care. A single excessive dose of these glycosides invariably results in death from cardiac paralysis in a short time."[1]

Paul D. White, who considers digitalis one of the most valuable drugs in heart disease, nevertheless pointed out that "auricular paralysis, auricular fibrillation, various high grades of heart-block, a coupled rhythm due to ventricular premature beats every second beat, idioventricular rhythm, ventricular paroxysmal tachycardia, and ventricular fibrillation have all been induced in man or in animals by massive doses of digitalis," and then goes on to say:

"When any of these disorders of cardiac mechanism are found to result from the digitalis given and not primarily from other factors, the drug should be discontinued, for a high percentage (50% to 90%) of the lethal dose has probably been given by the time such disorders are found."[2]

Thienes and Haley referring to digitalis mention that "the chief site of the toxic action is on the heart muscle

[1] *JAMA,* June 5, 1948.
[2] P. D. White, *Heart Disease.*

and that prolonged or severe poisoning causes fragmentation of heart muscle fibers, with areas of necrosis (degeneration, death) scattered throughout the heart."[3]

Levine stated "that while therapeutic doses of digitalis produce no pathological changes in the heart muscle, toxic doses do cause definite necrosis (death, degeneration) of the heart muscle fibers and inflammatory changes and also changes in brain cells."[4]

Doctors know that digitalis is a poison, but nonetheless consider it a most valuable remedy for those who suffer from congestive heart failure. To avoid the damage that may result from its use, they prescribe it in therapeutic doses which according to Levine average "about 35 to 40 percent of the lethal (deadly) dose."

The basic fallacy in this explanation is the fact that digitalis, like most other drugs, tends to accumulate in the system, and that its damaging effects are usually not recognized in the early stages since as White pointed out "a high percentage (50 to 90%) of the lethal dose probably has been given by the time such disorders are found."

The U. S. Dispensatory points out that "at times when the drug is being used continuously, no evidence of its action may be manifest for several days and then suddenly symptoms of toxic effects come on. This is what is meant by the term cumulative action."

Thienes and Haley state that its "prolonged use leads to poisoning" and that "the action of impounded digital can be demonstrated as late as two weeks after the last dose."

When a physician is confronted with a heart case, he is often in a great dilemma. He must do something to help the patient and where digitalis is indicated, he will resort to it as the best possible remedy at his disposal even though he knows that it is toxic. In his effort to be as careful as possible, he may use one digitalis preparation in preference to another on the assumption that it may be less poisonous. However, this is a delusion since the degree of effectiveness of a digitalis preparation is directly proportionate to its degree of toxicity and a digitalis preparation is only less poisonous when the body fails to absorb it.

[3] Thienes and Haley, *Clinical Toxicology.*
[4] Levine, *Clinical Heart Disease.*

Levine confirmed this by writing that "confusion has resulted because absorption of these preparations varies considerably when given orally."

And White emphasized this fact even more strongly by stating "that the toxic and therapeutic effects of various preparations of digitalis or of other drugs of the digitalis series are parallel; a preparation that can be taken in large dosage without toxic effects is apt likewise to be therapeutically inactive and a preparation that is very active therapeutically tends quickly to cause toxic symptoms."

Because of the poisonous effect of the digitalis preparations, some authorities have in recent years become more partial to the preparation known as digitoxin, on the assumption that this preparation is less poisonous. That this is an illusion is affirmed by Masters who pointed out that "the symptoms of digitoxin poisoning . . . do not differ from poisoning with other types of digitalis," and furthermore, "since digitoxin has a definite cumulative action, the toxicity persists longer than after other preparations of digitalis."

When the heart is in failure, it is dilated and cannot contract properly. This results in many instances, in shortness of breath, swelling of the ankles, retention of fluid in the system with danger of impending collapse.

Digitalis, in these cases, often provides dramatic relief. Its use slows down the heart and brings about a deeper contraction of the muscle. But since the drug is of a poisonous nature, one can very well realize how dangerous its use can ultimately become.

It is true that when used in moderate doses, the degenerative effects of this drug may not be apparent for some time. Its cumulative effect, however, is unavoidable and when used over a period of time, can easily lead to an increase in the degenerative changes in the heart.

Furthermore, its effect varies with the individual case. David P. Barr,[5] after pointing out that in digitalis "only a narrow margin separates therapeutic and toxic dosage," mentioned that because of oversimplification of dosage, the prevalence of rapid digitalization, and intravenous administration, "the dangers of the drug appear to be greater now

[5] "Hazards of Modern Diagnosis and Therapy—The Price We Pay," *JAMA*, December 10, 1955.

than ever before," and then pointed out that the age of the patient, the degree of the heart failure, and the use of other medications in the case, make the heart "more susceptible to the action of the drug," and are also to a great degree implicated in "the variable responsiveness" that takes place.

One can well understand why the cautious physician reduces the dosage of this drug to a mere "maintenance dose" as rapidly as possible, and dispenses with its use as soon as he can.

The Mercurial Diuretics

Next to digitalis, come the diuretics or the drugs which excite an increased elimination of fluid through the kidneys. The drugs most popularly used for this purpose are the mercurials, such as salyrgen, mercupurin and mercuhydrin.

In congestive heart failure, the heart is unable to keep up with its work and this often causes the feet to swell and the abdomen and lungs to fill up with fluid. Salyrgen, mercuhydrin and mercupurin injected into the body, force the expulsion of large quantities of fluid through the kidneys. This relieves the heart of the added strain and protects it against the danger of collapse.

However, here too it is important to bear in mind that these remedies can be quite dangerous and often cause additional damage or even collapse.

Dr. Leon Merkin, from the Cardiac Clinic of the City Hospital of New York, dealing with this subject, stated as follows:

"With the rapid growth in the number of cases in which mercurial diuretics have been administered, we find in the literature an increasing number of reports of untoward (adverse) effects resulting from the parenteral administration of these drugs. Among the side reactions the most important is the death of the patient shortly after the injection.

"Sudden death was not always the only side reaction to the injection of a mercurial diuretic. We find other less tragic reactions which, however, are also important," Dr.

Merkin stressed, and then as an illustration of how dangerous these drugs can be, described two cases in which collapse followed the use of this remedy.[6]

Tetany, uremia, not due to kidney or cardio-vascular disease but due to the use of these drugs, fever, and in some cases, stupor are some of the serious side-reactions which occur from the use of these drugs.

"One may wonder why these side-reactions and death . . . are comparatively rare even though the number of injections reaches thousands per day," Dr. Merkin asked, and then replied, "The answer is that side-reactions are much more frequent than doctors suspect. Very often these reactions are transient, and at the same time the clinical picture is obscured by other signs and symptoms arising from the heart failure.

"Without knowledge of the bio-chemical shift which can occur after administration of a mercurial, the signs and symptoms of the side-reaction will either not be heeded, or they will be attributed to quite different causes and wrongly interpreted," Dr. Merkin concluded.

Dr. Merkin pointed out that the administration of the mercurials leads among other things, to the excretion of many other essential elements, to a "diminution of the alkalinity of the body, thus promoting acidosis, which is further increased by simultaneous use of acidifying diuretics, e.g., ammonium chloride," to a disturbance in the balance between sodium and potassium leading to a preponderance of potassium in the system.

On this point, Dr. Merkin pointed out that "potassium intoxication results in widespread impairment of neuro-muscular function" and that the "accumulation of potassium in the body causes mortality and morbidity."

An editorial in the *Journal of the American Medical Association* published November 17, 1951, stressed that "although congestive failure itself predisposes to thrombosis (a closing of a blood vessel) there is some evidence that this tendency is aggravated by currently accepted therapy for congestive failure and particularly by the injudicious use of mercurial diuretics," and then quotes the finding of March and Pere, Russel and Zohuam, as well

---

[6] "Untoward Effects of Treatment with Mercurial Diuretics," *N. Y. State Journal of Medicine,* Oct. 15, 1949.

as the more recent findings of Marvel and Shullenberger, to prove this fact.[7]

Henry A. Schroeder, in a report read before the intern session of the American Medical Association, while stating that the mercurial diuretics arc of great value, nevertheless went on to say that their use may lead to an excessive elimination of sodium chloride as well as other essential elements, and that "this can lead to serious consequences if not recognized." He stated further that this drug is sometimes excreted rather slowly, and ended by saying that "the rather slow excretion of mercury can lead in certain subjects to the accumulation of toxic amounts."[8]

Flaxman, referring to the mercurial diuretics used in heart disease pointed out that "cases of sudden death due to the use of these drugs and fatal mercurialism continue to be reported."[9]

Boyd's remark in his chapter on "Necrosis of the Liver" that "the introduction of the newer diuretics, such as the organic mercury compounds in association with ammonium chloride, has diminished the dangers of ascites (swelling) as a cause of death, only to bring into greater prominence that of hemorrhage" is rather significant in connection with this point.[10]

The Nitrites

The nitrites (nitroglycerin and amylnitrate) relieve the severe angina attacks most dramatically. You just place a pellet of nitroglycerin under your tongue or break one of the tablets of amylnitrate in your handkerchief and presto, the attack subsides.

How do these remedies provide relief? They force the heart to work harder and help to dilate the arteries, and this lowers the blood pressure and relieves the attack.

However, it is imperative that we realize that no matter how welcome the relief may be, the basic condition has not changed. Furthermore, it is important to mention that

---

[7] "Thromboembolism Following Diureses."

[8] *Journal of the American Medical Association*, Nov. 17, 1951.

[9] "Drug Fatalities," *JAMA*, September 29, 1951.

[10] *Pathology of Internal Diseases*.

as the use of these remedies is continued, the attacks often recur with only more frequency and greater severity.

We have seen many sufferers from angina who started with one nitroglycerin tablet taken occasionally, but who ultimately ended up by taking them as often as every 15 minutes. Doctors know that nitrites, the same as other drugs, by combining with the oxygen, often actually cut down the availability of oxygen for the body and that this establishes a vicious cycle.

Now, if these drugs are inadvisable, what should be done to obviate the need for them? Our first objective is to restore a better circulation to the heart, and to overcome the periodic spasms which cause these attacks. While there is no single or stereotyped program which can be applied in all cases alike, we wish to point out that a program which embodies the use of simple, natural, easily digestible foods, and a restricted dietary regimen, even complete abstinence from food for limited periods of time when necessary, plus plenty of rest, often works wonders in these cases. Where drugs have been used over an extensive period of time and cannot be entirely withdrawn, a change to this kind of regimen will diminish the need for them and in time enable us to dispense with them completely in most instances.

This is a sound approach and should be followed in all types of heart disease. In those cases where digitalis and the mercurial diuretics have been used routinely and where, because of the condition of the patient, they cannot be discontinued immediately or completely, this basic approach helps to strengthen and rebuild the damaged and weakened heart and reduces the need for them, in many cases, may ultimately make their use entirely unnecessary.

We have seen many cases where mercurial diuretics were used as often as two or three times a week, but where by eliminating food for short periods of time and reducing the fluid intake, plus the application of the nursing care outlined in this book, the need for them was considerably reduced or the patient was enabled to do without them altogether.

Drugs Which Influence the Blood Clotting Mechanism

In coronary thrombosis or any other condition in which the blood congeals and forms clots, dicoumarol and heparin are used to thin the thickened blood. These drugs accomplish this by reducing the production of the blood clotting elements or by interfering with their normal effects on the blood.

That such methods are dangerous is well known. They can cause various blood derangements, lead to hemorrhage, and have caused many deaths. Flaxman[11] pointed out that dicoumarol accounted for eleven fatal hemorrhages bringing the total so far recorded from this drug to thirty-two. These fatalities resulted even where there was careful laboratory control "and despite long prior use without serious complications."

He further pointed out that many cases of non-fatal reactions have been reported from the use of this drug, and quoted Link, the developer of this drug (to the effect), "That the briefest meditation on the strictly theoretical aspects of the clotting phenomena leaves one with the appalling feeling that tampering with the coagulability of the blood is hazardous business."

Incidentally, it is well to mention at this point that many of the drugs used in the treatment of disease can influence the coagulability of the blood to a profound degree.

Dr. Harry Gold, well-known New York heart specialist, in a discussion of the action of drugs on the blood pointed out that "a dose of pilocarpine, muscarine or barin can nearly double the white cell count in the circulating blood," that "a dose of epinephrine can cause a fairly pronounced increase in the red cell count," and "can increase the coagulability of the blood from 200 to 300 percent."

He also stated that "chloroform can produce an almost complete disappearance of the coagulability of the blood," and that phenylhydrazine and its derivatives, antipyrine and aminopyrine, acetanilid and acetophenetidin and the

[11] "Drug Fatalities," *Journal of the American Medical Assn.,* Sept. 29, 1951.

sulfanilamides influence the health of the blood in different ways.[12]

Of course, it is important that to obtain results, the thickened blood be thinned, but it is one thing when this is accomplished by following a regimen which helps bring about this change naturally, and quite another when it is done with a remedy which tampers "with the coagulability of the blood."

Some years ago, Dr. Ernest Klein, a physician from Europe, connected with New York University, Bellevue Medical Center, disclosed that a diet of orange juice diluted in water will help thin the thickened blood.[13] Dr. Klein was subsequently discharged from his position in the hospital, apparently because he published the results of his findings without obtaining prior approval from his medical colleagues.

Levine stated that "the diet during the early days (of an attack) should be confined to liquids, gradually returning to more ordinary food in small amounts," and then mentioned that "it has been advised that a low calorie diet (500 to 800 calories a day) should be used in acute coronary thrombosis and, in fact, is being advocated in the treatment of any severe or stubborn case of congestive heart failure," pointing out further that "this semi-starvation diet diminishes the work of the heart, and produces other favorable effects on the circulatory dynamics."[14]

If in addition to a low calorie intake, we also make sure that the food is easily digestible and provides the body with its much needed minerals, vitamins and enzymes, and when, in addition to this, we also provide the other care which helps to restore normal functioning, we do everything possible to counteract the progress of the disease and thin the thickened blood.

That abstinence from food for short periods of time and restriction of the fluid intake is of great help in these cases, is recognized by many outstanding authorities. Many physicians are acquainted with the dramatic results obtained by the Karrell diet consisting merely of seven ounces of milk used four times a day.

12 *Journal of the American Medical Assn.*, August 3, 1940.
13 *New York Medicine*, May 1949.
14 *Clinical Heart Disease.*

Levine in discussing the efficacy of the Karrell diet explains that "semi-starvation produces a fall in blood pressure, in pulse rate and in the basal metabolic rate," and that "this may diminish the work of the heart and may thereby improve the circulation when failure is present."

Continuing on the same subject, Levine quotes Proger who suggested "that patients suffering from severe heart failure be kept on a diet containing adequate protein but only 500 to 800 total calories," and that such diets be continued for months, possibly indefinitely.

Dr. Irving C. Cutter, in one of his syndicated articles, related that J. Hatsilver, after trying numerous types of management, finally decided to place forty-eight of his high blood pressure cases on a bold starvation program. Each patient was kept on nothing but fruit juices, tomato juice, hot lemonade or vegetable broth for six days. On the seventh day, he was given a normal diet. This program was repeated each week as long as the symptoms improved, or until the blood pressure was reduced to normal.

Relief of symptoms in 90 percent of the cases was "dramatic," Dr. Cutter wrote. "Headaches and sleeplessness disappeared within three days, and dizziness, shortness of breath, and other symptoms were usually relieved by the end of the first week. In certain instances, the period of reduced pressure was fairly extensive and a number of otherwise incapacitated patients returned to full or part time employment."[15]

We have demonstrated the efficacy of this approach in some of the most difficult cases. In describing some of these cases, we do not mean to imply that no recoveries occur in standard practice, but merely how much more complete the results would be if sound physiological methods were employed in these cases.

[15] *Daily News,* October 8, 1935.

CHAPTER XVII

CASE HISTORIES

The Case of Mr. S.

Mr. S. is a case in point. Mr. S. was 59 years old. He had been sick for a long time, but the family decided to resort to the hygienic treatments when the doctors who attended his case held out no hope for his recovery and said that death was merely a matter of days.

As soon as we stepped into the sick room, we realized that we were dealing with a very sick man. Mr. S. was lying there all propped up with pillows, gasping for breath, his face flushed with a deep bluish hue. An examination revealed an extremely enlarged and damaged heart and extensive circulatory damage. His legs were badly swollen and his abdomen and part of his chest were filled with fluid. He had great difficulty in passing his urine, voiding only small quantities at a time.

A physician, who was connected with one of New York's large hospitals and who was regarded as an excellent heart man, performed the examination.

"What do you think of his chances for recovery?" we asked the physician after he had completed his examination and we had stepped into another room. "This man may die within the next 24 hours; but whether he dies tonight or tomorrow, there isn't much that can be done for him," he replied.

Because of this seemingly hopeless situation, and because all that could possibly have been done by medicine had been tried, the physician was willing to try the rational approach. We started by eliminating all food and by discontinuing all medication. All that we permitted for the first three days was about two ounces of freshly squeezed orange or grapefruit juice about every two or three hours. Warm cleansing enemas and hot mustard foot baths were used twice daily.

To keep a check on how his kidneys were functioning, we left instructions that the family collect his urine and keep a record of his daily output.

We need not mention that the first few days were most trying. The first hopeful sign came when the patient began to pass large quantities of urine many times the amount of liquid he was taking in.

Before long, several significant changes became noticeable. His breathing became easier, deeper, and more regular. His face and skin began to lose their sickening bluish hue, changing to a paler, healthier color. He was able to rest more comfortably and sleep much better.

As these improvements continued, our patient began to clamor for food. We began with small servings of grapefruit and oranges, but later added other fruits in small quantities.

A few days later we started with small meals, served at regular intervals; grapefruit and raw grated apple or stewed prunes for breakfast, lettuce and tomato salad with a small portion of a plain steamed vegetable for lunch, and a similar meal for dinner.

A few days later, we added other raw vegetables to his salad and also increased his meals by adding small portions of cottage or pot cheese for lunch and a baked potato for dinner.

An orange or portions of grapefruit were permitted between meals when he was hungry.

Later, some rye krisp or shredded wheat was added to his breakfast, and small servings of chicken, lamb chop or fish twice or three times a week were permitted in place of the cottage or pot cheese.

It took about four weeks before Mr. S. was able to get out of bed. We first sat him up in bed for short periods of time, with his feet dangling down. A few days later he was able to get into a chair, sitting up a half hour at first, gradually increasing the time each day. Later we encouraged him to take a few steps, increasing the distance with each day. Finally he was strong enough to move about from one room into the other.

His treatments commenced about the middle of March.

He lived on the top floor and by the time the warm weather set in, he was able to walk up to the roof for fresh air and sunshine, remaining there at first for about an hour, gradually increasing the time.

His progress was slow but steady. He continued to grow stronger and after six or seven months, he had sufficiently recovered to be able to return to work.

About eight years later, we were again called to see him. This time because he suffered a mild stroke. He was then about 67 years old. He had continued at his work since his original recovery until this happened. After about two and a half or three months of the same type of care, Mr. S. was again able to return to his job.

We were called to see him once more when he was about 72 years old, about fourteen years after we had first treated him for his congestive heart failure. Again we found him suffering from difficult breathing, swollen legs and abdomen, and again he had difficulty passing his urine.

Members of his family expressed the opinion that worry because of the induction of his grandson into the Armed Services undoubtedly contributed to his breakdown this time.

A short fast followed by a carefully regulated program plus good nursing care and rest in bed brought about sufficient improvement to enable him to get out of bed and finally go outdoors for short periods of time, but could not completely clear up the swelling of his ankles and feet.

The family, hoping that medical care might bring added improvement, then decided to call in a physician who administered a variety of drugs. Results were disappointing, however, and the patient died a few months later. By that time the family accepted his death as a welcome relief since they felt that his lingering existence caused him a great deal of misery.

"Frankly we expected him to die years ago and never thought that he would have so many more years of good life," was his wife's comment at that time.

While physiologically correct methods have proven highly successful in these cases, it is imperative that the care be supervised by one who is skilled in the application of these methods, since the neglect of even one minor factor may defeat our objective.

The question is not merely one of controlling the food intake or of providing enough rest, but of making sure that every little detail that enters into the management of a case of this kind be carefully controlled.

We Fail to Face Facts

Consciously or unconsciously many people go on deceiving themselves. It seems easier this way, and like the proverbial ostrich, they persist in ignoring the realities. At the time this book was first published our nation was greatly upset by the report of President Eisenhower's heart attack. To most people this came as a terrific shock since the President had regular checkups and was always reported to be in fine condition. The *U. S. News & World Report* in its September 23, 1955, issue, stated that while the numerous reports "about the President's good appearance and robust health" made some people wonder whether these reports might not have been deliberately exaggerated, the fact was that President Eisenhower was "in peak condition," while *The New York Times,* September 27, 1955, pointed out that a checkup on August 1, 1955, "failed to detect any hint of arterial disease."

And yet, a coronary attack does not develop suddenly. We keep building up to it, and a superficial appearance of what is usually regarded as robust health is not an indication that a heart condition may not be developing.

Dr. Paul Dudley White, called in consultation on the President's case, rightly stated that while it is not always easy "to diagnose the thickening of a coronary artery before an attack" *(it)* (the hardening) "may occur years before the thrombosis."

This disease is "about the commonest important illness that besets a middle-aged man in this country today," Dr. White pointed out and added that "the average age is about fifty in this condition." Since the President's age was nearing 65, he was "fifteen years ahead of the game from the standpoint of that type of illness."

We were pleased to note that Dr. White, in replying to what causes the disease, specified stress and strain, diet, alcohol and tobacco among the factors which might contribute to its development. However, we couldn't but wonder why, if the onset of this disease is to be controlled or checked, aren't these factors stressed ahead of time, as a measure of prevention?

Because of the President's illness, coronary artery disease has recently become a subject of wide discussion, and scientific writers continue to quote authorities to the effect that the disease is not nearly as dangerous now as it was in the past, and that a greater number of cases recover now from their attacks than formerly.

We should all be grateful for this, but an investigation will disclose that whatever progress has been made in this direction has taken place not because of any new remedies, but because there has been a vast improvement in the handling of these cases, more in line with the approach advocated in this book.

We note from the press that the President took no food except orange juice for the first few days, and then was kept on a much more careful diet. The use of oxygen is, of course, standard procedure and was necessary in the President's case. But we still ask, why weren't the factors enumerated by Dr. White as possible causes of hardening checked before the heart attack set in to prevent the existing condition to end up in a heart attack.

President Eisenhower died at the age of 78, about thirteen years after his first heart attack. Soon after, in 1957, he suffered a stroke, and this was later followed by two heart attacks in 1965 and four heart attacks in 1968. During these years he also suffered from a variety of other ills. In 1956, he was operated for ileitis, he had his gall bladder removed in 1966, and a month before his death he was operated upon for an intestinal obstruction, which was subsequently followed by pneumonia.

Nobody can be certain how long President Eisenhower could have lived, but we are positive his life could have been extended considerably as much of the misery and suffering that he went through in later years could have been avoided if the care outlined in this book would have been adopted immediately after his first heart attack and would have been consistently followed. It would have provided the necessary protection against his future heart attacks and would have strengthened his body sufficiently to protect it against the other disorders that developed later.

Arthur and His "Cup of Tea"

Not only do we deceive ourselves by refusing to face facts, we also deceive ourselves when we blame a sudden attack on something that has taken place or has been done just before the attack, conveniently overlooking the many "overt" acts which have been building up to it over a period of many years.

Some years ago, we were called to see a man who was rushed to the hospital because he suddenly "went blind." It was during the hot summer months and this man, like millions of others, spent the day preceding the attack at a favorite beach, and while there, ate one or two frankfurters on rolls.

Now millions of others like him visited the beach and partook of the same type of frankfurters without any apparent ill effects, but, since the attack happened so soon after he ate the frankfurters, what other logical reason could there be except that the frankfurters poisoned him and caused his blindness?

Hemorrhages resulting from a rupture of the hardened blood vessels of the eyes actually caused his blindness, but he had no inkling that he was suffering from this condition and that he had been building up to it over a long period of time.

We have known Arthur for many years, and his collapse did not come as a surprise to us. He was extremely overweight with a large protruding abdomen. His sickly greyish complexion and his catarrhal condition have been part of him as long as we could remember. Whenever one saw him, he would be eating something. He would finish a meal in one home, then visit another home and sit down to another full meal all over again. He would eat indiscriminately and never seemed to have enough.

He kept harking back to the one or two frankfurters that he had eaten on the day preceding the attack, but conveniently forgot or did not wish to remember, the thousands of frankfurters and the countless meals of rich and indigestible food which he had eaten all through life.

181

Somewhere, a story is being told about a lady who while on her summer vacation ate a very hearty meal, asking for double portions of some of her favorite dishes, finally finishing her meal with a cup of tea. When, soon after her meal, she developed a severe stomach attack, she blamed it all on the last cup of tea. The frankfurters in Arthur's case were apparently his "cup of tea."

Some of you may wonder what the final outcome was in this case. For years, Arthur refused to pay attention to our warnings, but this collapse made him realize that if he was to get well, a drastic change was imperative. He, therefore, insisted that he be taken out of the hospital and be moved to a place where he could obtain our type of care. In compliance with his wishes, he was moved to a private sanitarium where our program was carried out without any difficulties.

We started by withholding all food, permitting only sips of water when thirsty, made use of cleansing, warm water enemas and hot mustard foot baths to promote better elimination and improve the circulation.

Three days later, we started feeding him small quantities of freshly squeezed orange or grapefruit juice every two hours, reducing the enemas and foot baths to one a day.

It didn't take long before the first signs of improvement began to appear. He began to lose weight, his blood pressure began to come down, and his heart began to function much more strongly and more regularly.

About a week or ten days later, we added some solid food. Raw and stewed fruits, small servings of raw grated vegetables, some steamed vegetables and an occasional baked potato, made up his meals. Later, we included small portions of cottage cheese twice a week.

Salt, butter, sugar, cream, milk, coffee, tea, bread, cereals, sauces, meat, eggs, puddings, as well as all fried and fat foods were strictly excluded.

Before long, the frequency of the enemas was again reduced, first to one every other day, then to one every third day, and finally they were discontinued altogether.

As he continued to improve, we were able to substitute the full epsom salt bath for the mustard foot bath. We continued this program for about three or four months.

During this time, he lost a considerable amount of weight, his heart became much stronger, his blood pressure came down to about 160, his kidneys were doing their work more efficiently, while the hemorrhages in the eyes were almost completely reabsorbed.

While his vision was still somewhat blurred, it had improved sufficiently to enable him to return to a fairly normal existence.

By the time he left his sick bed, he weighed about forty pounds less, and his loosely hanging clothes and sagging muscles showed what he had been through. The important thing, however, was that his blood pressure had been considerably reduced, his heart was again able to do its work, and his vision had come back practically to normal.

Nick N., the Man Who Wanted to Die

That hardening of the arteries often leads to loss of vision is well known. Another case involving loss of vision is the case of Nick N.

Nick N. was only forty years old when he lost his sight. His illness began with sharp pains in his head and in his extremities which persisted without relief for several months.

While under the care of his doctors, Nick began to notice that his vision was gradually growing dimmer, becoming increasingly worse with time. At the suggestion of the doctors, he agreed to go to a hospital where a few days later, he lost his sight completely.

Repeated checkups disclosed that he was suffering from a condition known as acute toxic neuro-retinitis, which was brought on by hardening of the arteries and possible kidney damage.

Members of the family were told by the doctors that though Nick was still a relatively young man, the damage to his eyes resulted from deteriorations in his body equalling those found in a seventy-year old man, and that no hope for the recovery of his vision could be held out.

In search for help, the family brought Nick to New York. He was taken to a private hospital where a well known New York physician only confirmed the previous findings. An eye specialist called in to examine his eyes, reported the loss of almost the entire vision of his left eye, and loss of the greater part, especially the central part, of his right eye.

Since neither the general practitioner nor the eye specialist was able to offer any concrete help, these doctors had no objection to the use of our unorthodox approach, even though they were clearly skeptical of results.

As a first step, all food and all drugs were eliminated. Nick was put to bed and was fed nothing but a few mouthfuls of orange juice or grapefruit juice several times a day.

In addition, warm cleansing enemas and hot baths were ordered twice daily, after which he was wrapped in wet sheets to induce sweating. His eyes were kept covered to exclude all light, while the room was darkened for further protection.

This program was carried through for about a week. Then some solid food was introduced. Firstly, sliced oranges and grapefruit, later small meals of fresh fruits and raw vegetables. The enemas and hot baths were reduced to once a day.

Hospitals, as a rule, are not suitable places to put such a regimen into operation since it is usually impossible to obtain the food we order and since the nurses and other members of the staff are not trained to follow this kind of routine. One may wonder, therefore, how we were able to put this regimen into operation.

As a matter of fact, none of the workers in the hospital were aware of what was actually going on. The enemas and the baths were administered upon doctor's orders. Nothing was mentioned in the chart about his diet. The nurse would bring in his tray, and when she left the room, one of the relatives who was always with him during the day, ate the food. The fruit juices and the the other foods which he was to eat were brought in by the family from the outside.

It is only proper to mention that we had no way of telling how badly damaged his eyes were and therefore, could not tell how much we could accomplish. In cases of this kind, recovery is always limited by the degree of damage, and only the tissues which are not fully destroyed have a chance of being restored to health. Where reabsorption of the hemorrhage or the exudates is delayed, or where the inflammatory condition persists over an extended period of time, degenerative changes may progress to the point where irreversible damage sets in, precluding all chances of recovery.

It was fortunate for Nick that his condition was of comparatively recent origin, and that no really destructive changes had taken place in his eyes, but we had no way of determining this at first.

At the start, Nick was terribly despondent. He had never been seriously ill before, and the thought that he might never see again was almost unbearable to him. If he couldn't see again, life wasn't worth living and he would rather die!

Over and over again, the patient would keep on asking whether he would ever see again. We could not be sure, but telling him this would have been like pronouncing his death sentence. So while the members of his family were apprised of our doubts, the patient was constantly assured that everything would come out all right.

So far as his general condition was concerned, improvement began to show almost immediately. His blood pressure began to drop almost from the start of the treatment and continued to drop until it reached a normal level. As far as his sight was concerned, however, no discernible improvement was apparent during the first ten days or two weeks.

Nick reached the depth of despair. We kept telling him that he must have patience, but so far as he was concerned, life was not worth living. Life without his sight was worthless. Unless he regained his eyesight, he would kill himself!

Then early one morning as he awakened from sleep and opened his eyes, he seemed to notice the shadow of two horses reflected from the street on the wall opposite his bed. Unbelievingly he turned to look at other things. No, it was not a trick of the imagination—he was actually able to see again.

Exultantly, he began to shout, "I can see! I can see!"

At first his vision was dim and blurred. He was able to distinguish only outlines, but this change was enough to imbue him with new hope. Now he knew that his sight was coming back!

Improvement continued with each day. About a week

185

later, Nick left the hospital and was taken to his sister's home where he stayed until he had fully recovered.

We need not mention how surprised the eye specialist was when upon re-examination a few weeks later (March 30, 1946), he found that the condition had completely cleared up. The following is a copy of his final report on the case:

"Mr. Nick N. shows almost complete regression of the neuro-retinitis. His vision is R. 20/25; L. 20/30 and he accepts no correction. The tension is normal, lenses and media are clear. The fundi show minute whitish soft retinal exudates, mostly in the posterior poles. There are also some radiating yellowish lines in the macular region which are probably the remains of the retinal edema, surrounding the macula. No hemorrhages are present; the disc margins are sharp and the color of the disc is normal except for a slight yellowish pallor temporally. The retinal spots are more numerous in the left than in the right eye. On examining his left fundus with a binocular Gullstrand ophthalmoscope, the whitish exudates appeared to be in the nerve fibre layers of the retina.

"The peripheral fields were normal. The blind spots showed slight enlargement which, however, is of no consequence. There were no other scotomata present."

When we compare this report with the one of only a few weeks before, February 17, 1946, which stated that the examination revealed the loss of almost the entire vision of his left eye and the greater part, especially the central part of his right eye, and that the pathology, limited to the fundi showed nasal blurrings of both discs, numerous exudates and flame-shaped hemorrhages in the retina, mostly of the posterior pole, and cholesterol deposits in the deeper layers of the retina, we can see how remarkable his recovery was.

Nick continued his treatment for another three months, and then returned to his home town and resumed his former work.

An interesting highlight in connection with Nick's recovery was the fact that while before his illness, he was nearsighted and had to wear glasses, the examination by the eye specialist revealed that he was able to discard his glasses completely.

Unfortunately, not all cases respond alike. As stated

before, the results depend upon the extent of the damage, and in cases where the exudates and hemorrhages are not quickly absorbed and the inflammatory condition is not quickly eliminated, the damage may become irreversible.

This is the reason it is so important that no suppressive treatments be used and that the measures employed in these cases help to normalize function and repair the damage as rapidly as possible.

The Case of Mrs. G.

In many years of practice, we have been confronted by many so-called "hopeless" cases of heart and blood vessel disease which made phenomenal recoveries by following our type of care. We recollect the case of Mrs. G. who was under our care about thirty years ago. Mrs. G. was suffering from the after-effects of a coronary thrombosis and complained of excruciating angina attacks which came on at regular intervals.

Here, too, we were called in as a last resort, and here, too, the opinion of the physician who examined her is of interest.

"If I were you, I wouldn't touch her. Why put your head into a sick bed. And besides, she is Dr. M's patient." (Here he mentioned the name of a well-known New York heart specialist), "and he will have your life if he finds out that you are meddling with his case," the physician cautioned us after the examination.

However, since we have been long accustomed to be called in on difficult cases, this was not a valid reason for refusing to take care of her.

"Nobody is able to do anything for her and with our treatment there is at least a chance," we replied, to which the physician had nothing to say.

We resorted to our usual procedure and Mrs. G. was under our care for about six months. By the end of that time she was completely free from pain and able to return to a fairly normal life. She surprised the heart specialist by visiting him after her recovery, and he wanted to know everything she had done to get well.

About seventeen years later, Mrs. G. came in to see us again. She was then about 72 or 73 years old and again in need of help. Years of neglect had made her sick again, and by this time her condition had again greatly deteriorated. That made matters even worse since she was no longer willing to cooperate.

The Progress of Mrs. M. G.

Even in cases where a great deal of the damage is irreversible, much can be done to stem the progress of the disease and to bring about improvement in health.

The case of Mrs. M. G. is a case in point. We will let Mr. G. tell the story of his wife in his own way:

"My wife suffered from stomach trouble even before we were married. Soon after our marriage she developed high blood pressure. Not long after, she began to complain of severe headaches and dizziness and pains all over her body. Doctors told us that this was due to hardening of the arteries.

"Following the suggestion of doctors, we took her to Saratoga Springs where the baths, plenty of rest, and the invigorating air made her feel much better. Encouraged by this, we returned to Saratoga Springs several seasons in succession.

"In 1931, a few weeks after our return from Saratoga Springs, her cousin died suddenly, and the shock of this made a ghost of her. She was then forty-eight years old and her blood pressure soared to 260, which could not be budged.

"We had to wait upon her hand and foot, and we kept a woman in constant attendance to take care of her.

"At that time somebody suggested that a change in diet might help her, and a doctor who specialized in this type of care prescribed a diet for her and taught her how to relax. From then on, an entirely new life began for her. She began to feel like a new woman. Her pains began to lessen almost immediately and in time disappeared altogether. Her appetite and digestion before long returned to normal. She became much stronger and her blood pressure showed a gradual reduction.

"At one time her vision became so bad that she couldn't cross the street without help. She thought she was losing her sight and became terribly frightened by it. The practitioner's encouragement and patient guidance helped her immeasurably at that time.

"Her vision gradually improved and she was able to resume her former activities.

"Because of the many years that she suffered from high blood pressure, her heart became badly damaged, but the program she followed strengthened the heart sufficiently to enable her to carry on her normal activities.

"On several occasions, especially during the latter years of her life, her heart would sometimes give way. Whenever this happened, this doctor's instructions helped to bring her around in quick order.

"My wife followed these instructions for the rest of her life. Before these treatments were started, no doctor could hold out any hope for her. This care and the patient guidance of her doctor not only relieved her pains but prolonged her life by many years.

"She passed away at the age of 70 as a result of a heart attack, and we know that this new way of living gave her many years of comfort and happiness."

To elaborate on this case, we wish to mention that the care in Mrs. G.'s case was similar in most respects to the care in the other cases we mentioned before. A careful nutritional regime, composed primarily of fresh fruits and vegetables, with small portions of easily digestible proteins; and simple natural treatments, gradually reduced her blood pressure from a high of about 250/140 to about 170/100.

Some years later, when, for a time, her vision became badly affected, complete rest and an especially restricted diet, in addition to simple natural care, gradually restored her sight sufficiently to enable her to lead a fairly normal life all over again.

CHAPTER XVIII

WHY THESE MEASURES ARE HELPFUL

The Usefulness of the Cleansing Enema

As you follow our approach in these cases, many questions will naturally arise, and among these would be why the different measures are employed.

You will notice that in almost every case the warm cleansing enema was used. The enema is practically a routine measure since it helps to eliminate the pressure and strain caused by gas and constipation.

Even a cursory examination will disclose that most sufferers from heart disease are constipated and suffer from gas pressure, and this condition exists even among those who have daily evacuations.

Dr. Harvey J. Kellogg of the Battle Creek Sanitarium pointed out that people who eat three meals a day and have only one evacuation daily suffer from intestinal stasis or sluggishness, while Dr. C. Ward Crampton, Chairman of Geriatrics, Medical Society of New York County, stated that "colonic delay of a week is possible for one with daily evacuation."[1]

When this condition exists, the patient is not only bothered with gas which presses up against the heart and aggravates the palpitation as well as the other heart symptoms, but often suffers from many other physical disorders such as a protruding abdomen, prolapsed organs, as well as mechanical pressure which affects the adjacent organs and hampers the circulation of the blood. It should be obvious that this throws an added burden upon the heart.

[1] "Young At Any Age," *Yearbook of N. Y. State Joint Legislative Committee on Problems of the Aging.*

Careful use of the enema helps to remove the accumulations in the colon and relieves the heart of the extra load caused by this condition.

The Reason for the Hot Baths

The full hot bath or the partial foot bath is used to promote elimination through the skin and kidneys, to improve circulation, and to promote relaxation.

Incidentally, different hot and cold applications can be used to great advantage to relieve many of the discomforts of heart disease. A cold compress applied over the heart goes a long way to check palpitation, while heat applied to the upper part of the back or between the shoulder blades counteracts pain in the chest and is of great help in heart and blood vessel spasms.

At this point we wish to stress the importance of keeping the feet warm. A hot water bottle, the electric pad, or the wearing of socks will be helpful for this purpose.

Why Control of Food Intake Is Helpful

We recommend partial or even complete abstinence from food for limited periods of time to rest the organs of digestion and give the organs of elimination a chance to catch up with their work of eliminating the undesirable by-products of metabolism from the body.

The value of small meals or abstemious eating is now generally recognized. It lessens the work of the digestive organs and reduces the work of the heart. We conserve the energies of the body when the work of all the organs of the body is reduced to a desirable and safe minimum.

Incidentally, it was only most recently that Dr. Clive McCay in a talk before The New York Academy of Medicine, pointed out that abstemious eating protects against the onset of the diseases of the heart and blood vessels.

Incidentally, this also explains why simple, easily digestible foods are important and why the foods which overburden the digestive organs must be eliminated.

Reason for Excluding Refined Grain Food Products

The reason we advocate the exclusion of refined grain food products should be self-evident. In these foods, all the essential protective elements, such as the vitamins, minerals and enzymes have been removed and very little has been left but the pure starch, the high carbohydrate content exclusive of all its vital elements. These foods not only fail to provide the body with indispensable vitamins, enzymes and minerals, they actually deplete the body of these essential protective elements, and this blocks or interferes with the assimilation of even good foods.

It is with good reason that these foods are often called the dead foods since modern refining and devitalizing processes remove most of their essential nutritive elements.

The Danger of the Concentrated Sugars

In our book *New Hope for Arthritis Sufferers,* we pointed out that sugar is a fuel and that when taken in concentrated form, it will feed the fires of the body too strongly and, as a result, actually waste energy and deplete our reserves even though on the surface they seem to provide a sense of exhilaration and well-being. Somogyi's explanation of how insulin disrupts the glandular balance in the body has proven the correctness of our conclusion.

When we stress the elimination of the concentrated sugars, we do not refer merely to the refined white sugar and white sugar products, but also to the concentrated natural sweets, such as the dried figs, dates, raisins, raw sugar and honey. At this point, we are not concerned with the protective elements which have been removed from the sugar when it has been refined and which are found in the natural sweets, but with the fact that excess sugar in any form ultimately depletes the energies of the body, although this may, at first, not be recognized.

It is imperative to stress at this point that a diet which would attempt to exclude all sugars, even if that were possible would be highly dangerous. Sugars are necessary to life, but we should obtain our sugars from fresh fruits, such as grapes, apples, pears, peaches, melons, the great variety of luscious berries, and the easily digestible root vegetables such as carrots, beets, parsnips, turnips, as well as the easily digestible starches like potatoes, corn, etc.

One of the dangers of concentrated sugar is that it overstimulates the pancreas and calls forth too much insulin. This often leads to a low blood sugar condition with its extreme debility. Ultimately this may so damage or exhaust the gland that diabetes may develop.

The Disadvantages of Coffee and Tea

You are undoubtedly aware by this time that to rebuild our depleted body, the reserves of the body must be rebuilt. This calls for a reduction in the expenditure of our energy to a bare minimum. We have reached the point of breakdown because we have recklessly squandered our reserves and if we are to replenish them, we must practice utmost economy in the use of the little that is still left in our body.

Coffee and tea, as well as all other stimulating indulgences are not only poor substitutes for the needed sustained energy, their use in the long run actually wastes a great deal of it.

Why Spices and Condiments Are Harmful

Spices and condiments are objectionable not only because they are irritating to the digestive system but because by stimulating the digestive glands, they whip up our jaded appetites and induce overeating.

This does not mean that our meals have to be monotonous, unsavory, or uninviting. However, to make our meals appetizing and enjoyable, we must spend at least as much time and thought in the preparation of these dishes as we do when preparing some of our conventional meals.

Tomatoes, leek, sweet onions, garlic, dill, sage, rosemary, caraway seeds, as well as lemon and honey carefully blended in with our foods, add most exotic flavors to our dishes and make our meals truly delicious.

Fresh air, sunshine, a congenial environment, emotional poise and good nursing care are other important requisites in these cases.

The Use of Oxygen

The oxygen used in the treatment of heart disease is a concentrated, irritating gas and not the same as the oxygen and nitrogen mixture we breathe. When used carelessly, it can cause harm. Nonetheless, when carefully employed in cases of heart failure, it often provides dramatic relief. We have seen many cases where its cautious use overcame the decompensation in the heart, rid the body of excess fluids, and made the elimination of mercurial diuretics, even in advanced cases of heart disease, possible.

Oxygen Therapy News, September 20, 1950, referred to Dr. R. L. Levy who pointed out that with the use of oxygen "pain is lessened or abolished, the heart rate falls, and respiration is slower and less labored. The patient is no longer restless. It is possible to curtail materially or stop entirely the use of opiates and sedatives."[2]

The above statement is in line with our findings and the fact that it helps to limit or eliminate the use of the opiates and sedatives only adds additional value to it.

Our primary aim should be to maintain our health so as to avoid lapsing into a condition where this therapy becomes necessary, but when this point is reached, the cautious use of oxygen can often save human life.

It should be needless to say that its application must be carefully supervised by one who is thoroughly experienced in the handling of these cases.

The handling of a heart case is not a simple matter. Many problems may arise which may require the decision of one skilled in the handling of these emergency measures.

However, to ensure gratifying results, it is imperative that the doctor or practitioner in charge of the case possesses a full grasp of the hygienic principles and understands how to make the delicate adjustments which are necessary to help the patient recover.

[2] *Bulletin,* New York Academy of Medicine, June 1950.

CHAPTER XIX

ADDITIONAL DISCUSSION ON
THE EFFECTS OF DRUGS

Hysteria, leading to unwarranted and often irresponsible claims, pervades not only the lay public but also respectable professional circles. Not so many years ago, Dr. Morris Fischbein, the then Secretary of the American Medical Association and Editor-in-Chief of the *Journal of the American Medical Association,* issued his little tract, "Syphilis, The Next Great Plague To Go," in which he claimed that one out of every ten Americans was suffering from syphilis and in need of the treatments then prevailing for this disease.

Aleta White, in a recent article in the *Saturday Evening Post,* described how a positive Wasserman blood test caused her to submit to treatments with the arsenical compounds, and what she has gone through as a result of it. She stated that an almost fatal reaction to the arsenic compounds made her deathly sick for months, and caused her severe skin conditions. Her tongue swelled up to the point where she could not swallow, while her face and cheeks puffed up and she looked like "a shapeless unrecognizable mass." She was almost blind for a time and often felt so miserable that suicide seemed the only way out.

She was finally saved when Dr. Joseph Earle Moore, Associate Professor of Medicine, Johns Hopkins University School of Medicine, submitted her to a newer more specific test which showed that she gave what is now called a biologic false positive reaction.

Lest you think that this may have been only an isolated instance, it is well to point out that Dr. Moore in his foreword to the article stated that the author was "one of several hundred persons I have observed and cared for professionally who at some time in the past have been falsely labeled with the diagnosis of syphilis."[1]

A rechecking of some of the claims made for the sulfa drugs, cortisone and ACTH, as well as for thousands of other drugs, which at one time or another have been offered to the ailing as a major solution to their health problems would make us blush with shame. No wonder the chemical path to health is strewn with disease and suffering. Publius was right when he stated that "there are some remedies worse than the disease," and our own Benjamin Franklin must have been aware of this when he stated that "he is the best physician who knows the worthlessness of most drugs."

The Dog Chasing His Tail

We know that sleeping pills can lead to addiction. This is true also of many other drugs. Any drug used with regularity ultimately leads to addiction and can cause untold damage.

Furthermore, the habitual use of many of these drugs make the patient so sensitive to pain that a condition which normally would be only mildly annoying becomes unbearable. This induces the use of larger doses or stronger drugs, leading only to more addiction.

The number of people who suffer from sleeplessness can be counted in the millions. Three hundred and fifty tons of barbiturates are used yearly in these cases in the United States according to *McCall's* magazine.[2] It should be evident that barbituarates do not provide natural sleep, and their habitual use only turns one into an addict.

Sleeplessness is merely a symptom of ill health and becomes aggravated when the underlying causes are not eliminated. It can be overcome only through the rebuilding of better health and the restoration of physical and mental relaxation. These changes rebuild a sound nervous system and restore normal, natural, restful sleep.

---

[1] "They Said I Had Syphilis," April 30, 1955.
[2] May, 1955.

The sufferer from heart disease needs an abundance of sleep; not the false, artificial sleep induced by drugs, but the sound, deep slumber which brings real relaxation and builds healthy nerves.

A Balance Between Rest and Physical Activities

Throughout this book you will note that the importance of rest is stressed. By rest we mean not only physical rest which is obtained by sleep and relaxation, but also physiological rest which we obtain when we reduce the work of the organs, so that they have a chance to rest and recuperate.

However, while physical and physiological rest are essential, the need for physical activities must not be overlooked. Life is synonymous with function. Too much inactivity induces stagnation and impairs the circulation. So while rest is essential, it must not be overdone. Both rest and exercise must be regulated in accordance with the needs of the individual case.

We stated before that unless the subject of drugs and their effect upon health is fully understood, a great deal of confusion may result.

The reason for this should be obvious. Our reliance upon drugs for the treatment of disease harks back thousands of years and is now standard practice. It should be made clear that unless the detrimental effects of drugs and the benefits that can be derived from the hygienic methods are fully understood, people may be at a loss to know what to do in case of disease.

To avoid this confusion, the question of the nature of disease and how sound physiological measures can be utilized for effective results must, therefore, be clearly understood. The individual must realize that our task is not merely to hold in check or suppress the symptoms of disease, but to eliminate the causes and promote the necessary bodily readjustments.

While we stress the harm that can result from a dependence upon drugs, it is well to point out that the trend toward a more constructive approach is rapidly gaining momentum, and that many new and helpful measures are coming into use. A perusal of present day medical literature will disclose that sound physiological concepts are rapidly coming to the fore.

We find no fault with those measures which enable the body to do an effective healing job, but we reject the measures which mask and suppress, since they hamper the body's efforts to make the necessary readjustments and restore lasting health. Furthermore, we find fault with any school of healing which overlooks the basic causes of disease and fails to promote basic physiological readjustments.

That sedatives, purges, stimulants, can be extremely harmful, is well known. They should be discontinued immediately. The medicines which are taken for the heart can also cause damage, but in some instances may have to be discontinued or tapered off more gradually depending upon the condition of the patient and the degree of damage. We are stressing this point again, since it is imperative to realize that these changes must be carefully supervised by one skilled in the handling of such cases and fully conversant with the application of the sound physiological approach.

CHAPTER XX

PHYSICAL EXERCISES AND
HEART DISEASE

That outdoor sports and physical exercises, when used in moderation, act as a valuable brake against the onset of heart disease is now being recognized by an ever greater number of authorities.

This does not mean that we can gorge ourselves on rich indigestible foods or that we can wear ourselves out in business or in our social activities and hope that long walks or a Sunday spent on the "greens" will undo the harm. It merely means that the outdoor life and physical exercises, indulged in properly and used in conjunction with the other wholesome habits of living, will provide a rounded out program of healthful living and serve as an added protection against the onset of these diseases.

Jean Mayer, Assistant Professor in the School of Public Health, Harvard University, in reporting on the physical fitness tests conducted by Dr. Hans Kraus and Mrs. Ruth Hirshland of the Institute of Physical Medicine, Bellevue Medical Center, pointed out that "several thousand American boys and girls attending public schools were compared to children of similar ages in Austria and Italy" and that the incidence of failure among our youngsters was 78.3 percent as against 8.5 percent for the European children.

He stated further that "the mortality from the so-called degenerative diseases, particularly heart disease, is exceptionally high among Americans between the ages of 35 and 55" and then mentioned that "accumulating evidence shows that lack of regular exercise is one of the factors involved."

We were glad to note that Jean Mayer mentioned that it

was merely *one* of the factors, since it is important that none of the other factors which play a part should be overlooked or disregarded. He stated it very aptly when he said "that our motorized mechanized 'effort saver' civilization is rapidly making us as soft as our processed foods, our foam rubber mattresses, and our balloon tires."[1]

Healthful Physical Exercises Helpful

Outdoor sports and physical exercises promote the intake of oxygen into the lungs, counteract stagnation, strengthen the abdominal muscles and increase the blood supply to the heart, and in this way do much to strengthen the heart and blood vessels.

Dr. Ernest Simonson, Associate Professor of Physiological Hygiene at the University of Minnesota Medical School, asserted that exercise enables the heart and lungs to handle large volumes of oxygen without strain and protects the nervous system against fatigue;[2] while Dr. Ernst Jokl, a leading European heart specialist who came to this country to set up a new Department of Clinical Physiology at the Valley Forge Heart Institute and Hospital, Fairview Village, Pa., commented on the fact that many athletes are in peak form and able to participate in competitive activities "long past the years when they would have been too old to compete a few generations ago," and pointed out that "one important explanation for this change is a life of healthful exercise."[3]

Dr. Julius Hofman, of Berlin and Bad Nauheim, when asked why the results obtained by exercise could not be obtained more simply and with equal certainty by drugs, mentioned that while "drugs enable the heart to utilize more of its available strength" (in other words, act as stimulants), it is not known "whether by continued use they increase the sum total of the heart's strength."

"But baths and gymnastics we know, by the way they influence the heart, increase its strength."[4]

[1] *New York Times Magazine Section,* Nov. 6, 1954; also graphically portrayed in *U. S. News,* March 19, 1954.

[2] *New York Times,* April 17, 1954.

[3] *New York Times,* March 20, 1953.

[4] *Remedial Gymnastics for Heart Affections.*

Points to Remember

Here are a few points which must be kept in mind in connection with physical exercise as it applies in heart diseases.

1. Never indulge in exercises indiscriminately. Make sure that you follow only those exercises which have been outlined for you to meet your particular needs.

2. A weak or debilitated person should exercise in a reclined position since this induces more complete relaxation and is least taxing to the heart.

3. Never exercise to the point of fatigue. Always stop before you are tired. If tired, stop, take deep, slow breaths, and rest, before you continue your exercises.

4. Avoid competitive sports.

5. Whenever possible, perform your exercises on a hard surface or on the floor.

6. All exercises should be done slowly.

Here are a few of the simpler exercises which strengthen the heart and the circulation, and benefit the body as a whole.

DEEP BREATHING EXERCISES

Abdominal Breathing Exercises

1. Lie down on hard surface or floor. Inhale slowly and deeply, expanding the abdomen as you breathe in. Then exhale slowly and completely, drawing your abdomen in. Inhale and exhale through nose, with mouth closed. Relax and repeat.

2. Repeat the same exercise with each nostril separately.

Chest Breathing Exercises

1. Take position as before. While inhaling through the nose, lift up your shoulders and collar bone, filling your chest with air, but the abdomen remains largely inactive.

2. Repeat the same exercise with each nostril.

A variation of these exercises is to lift and stretch your arms upward and above your head when inhaling, and to lower the arms when exhaling.

A modification of this exercise is to keep both arms at the sides, then raise them slowly to a horizontal position, when inhaling and return them to the sides when exhaling.

LEG EXERCISES

1. Assume reclining position and relax completely. Then, without bending your knees, raise both legs slowly as high as they will reach, then slowly lower them until they touch the floor. Make sure to do this exercise slowly and in an even manner. Relax, and repeat.

2. Repeat the same exercise with each leg separately.

The following exercises are permissible when the patient's strength returns; but we repeat that all exercises should be done only under careful direction.

SITTING-UP EXERCISES

Continue in reclined position and relax. Keeping the knees and legs straight, fully touching the floor, sit up slowly, stretching your arms and hands in front of you in an effort to touch your legs with your hands. Then slowly return to reclined position.

MORE ADVANCED LEG EXERCISES

1. Assume reclining position as in the simpler leg exercises, and relax. Then raise one leg slowly (knees straight), and when reaching the upright position, bend leg over first to the left side as far as it will reach; then to the right side as far as it will reach, then return to the center and lower leg to touch floor again.

2. Repeat the same movements with the other leg.

3. Repeat the same movements with both legs together, turning both legs first to one side then to the other side, then bringing them back to the center and lowering them until they touch the floor.

There are many other exercises which can be added as the patient regains his strength, but they should be done only under careful supervision.

STRETCHING EXERCISES

Stretching—Upward

Lie flat on your back and relax. Keep arms close to body. Then raise both arms slowly over your head and stretch—stretch—stretch. Return arms to side and repeat all over again.

Stretching Sideways (Upper Part of Body)

Lie flat on your back and relax. Bend upper part of trunk slowly to right side, then to left side. Return to normal position, rest and repeat.

Stretching Sideways (Lower Trunk)

Assume position as before. Bend lower part of trunk slowly first to right side then to left side. Return to straight position, rest and repeat.

Stretching Sideways (Whole Trunk)

Assume position as before. Keep arms close to body. Raise arms upward, then bend body to left, then to right and then return to normal position.

The Cradle Exercise

Raise both legs upward. Then as you lower your legs, raise upper part of body, rocking cradle fashion.

CHAPTER XXI

THE VALUE OF BATHS AND PACKS

We referred above to the benefits derived from the hot full bath or partial foot bath. Baths, wet packs, or compresses, as well as other forms of water treatment, are of great help in the diseases of the heart and blood vessels.

The hot bath relaxes the body, improves the circulation and promotes the elimination of toxins through the skin and kidneys. The full hot baths should be used when conditions permit, while foot baths should be resorted to in cases of extreme debility.

Hot packs and compresses applied locally have a softening and soothing effect and help to relax spasm and tension. They provide quick relief of pain.

Cool compresses have a soothing and calming effect, and are refreshing and invigorating.

You will notice that we mention the hot full bath or hot foot bath frequently in our case histories. Baths and compresses can be of great help when properly used. However, when used improperly or at the wrong time, they can overstimulate and increase debility. Make sure that the type of bath or application used in the case be carefully determined by the doctor or practitioner in charge.

It should be evident that the results in each case will vary, depending upon the degree of damage and the recuperative powers of the individual. However, we cannot stress too strongly the fact that, everything being equal, the best chances for recovery rest in a well planned nutritional program plus the care which aids the recuperative powers of the body to do an effective job of restoring the body to health.

It should not be difficult to see why such an approach can be so much more successful than a dependence on conventional methods. Our first task is to uncover the influences which have undermined the health of the patient and make sure that these deleterious influences are eliminated or checked.

Our second task is to institute a program which helps mobilize the body's curative forces so that maximum repair and restitution take place as rapidly as possible.

Our final task is to make sure that the program we follow helps in overcoming all systemic derangements which have contributed to the development of the diseased entity. This involves the rebuilding of digestion, the restoration of normal glandular function, the normalization of the blood, the improvement of the circulation, and the strengthening of the nervous system.

We are very much in agreement with Pottenger[1] who stated that in the treatment of the sick, we must endeavor to remove cause, restore disturbed function and establish nervous and psychic equilibrium.

Medicine in a State of Ferment

Medicine is in a state of ferment. Its leaders, research workers, and great numbers of its practitioners are becoming ever more aware of the hazards of medicine and are wondering how these hazards may be minimized or eliminated.

Dr. David P. Barr in a lecture read before the section on Internal Medicine at the 104th Annual Meeting of the American Medical Association, June 8, 1955, dealt with these hazards, and pointed out that accidents and misfortunes may result even when drugs are used "by conscientious and well informed physicians, earnestly trying to help their patients."

"One of the great hazards in the use of potent drugs is their inherent toxicity," Dr. Barr mentioned and quoted

[1] "Some Observations on Therapeutic Nihilism," *Medical Record*, September 10, 1927.

as an outstanding example digitalis in which "only a narrow margin separates therapeutic and toxic dosage."[2]

He further stated that the homeostasis of the body (the tendency to maintain the equilibrium of the internal environment), is strikingly changed or modified by a vast number of drugs and injections and pointed out that "no agent that can modify the internal environment or organic integrity of the body can be used without hazard."

He referred to the numerous side actions and toxic effects of the antibiotics and chemotherapy, and stressed the fact that "not all their potential dangers are immediately apparent"; mentioning further that there is sound reason for the inference that "past use of drugs may be responsible for the late appearance of symptoms or for the development of a chronic disease such as lupus erythematosus or periarteritis."

He continued by stating "It seems inevitable that with the increasing potency of drugs and the multitude of different reactions caused by single agents that there could be production of syndromes strikingly like those of previously known diseases," and then mentioned "that adverse action of drugs might be implicated in the pathogenesis (causes) of collagen diseases (diseases of a degenerative nature such as arthritis, hardening of the arteries, heart disease, rheumatic fever, etc.)."

Dr. Barr mentioned that more than 140,000 medications were available to practitioners in 1953, and that 90 percent of the drugs now in common use have been introduced within the last twenty-five years. In 1953 alone, 14,000 new preparations were added. Can you visualize what confusion and what havoc such a vast array of drugs can bring on?

Dr. Barr was careful to point out that in describing the dangers inherent in the use of drugs, he was not advocating therapeutic nihilism (the rejection of treatments). He need not. He can follow in the footsteps of Dr. Ray Lyman Wilburn, Dean Emeritus of Stanford University, who stated that "medicine based on pills and potions is becoming obsolete," and then pointed out that "those treat-

2 "Hazards of Modern Diagnosis and Therapy—The Price We Pay," *Journal of the American Medical Association,* December 10, 1955.

ments involving the use of heat, cold, water, electricity, movement and massage, having striking biologic reactions, including effects on psychic reactions, are more potent than many of the drugs gathered through many centuries by trial and error."[3]

Dr. Barr introduced the subject by quoting the dictum, "First of all, be sure you do no harm. *Primum non nocere."* It should be clear that only by avoiding the unpredictably dangerous drugs and by relying on sound, physiological measures of correction, can we live up to this dictum.

A point which must always be kept in mind is the fact that drugs often induce dangerous side-effects as well as unpredictable complications, and that many of the symptoms which are often attributed to the disease are in reality caused by the drugs used in the treatment of the disease.

The case of 79-year-old Mrs. G. is of interest in this connection. Mrs. G. is suffering from hypertensive heart disease and a severe form of hardening of the arteries.

She is now in fairly good condition, but only three months ago nobody would have thought that she could live. She was taking several kinds of medicine, was receiving injections of mercurial diuretics twice weekly, and from every point of view her condition was regarded as well-nigh hopeless.

She suffered from constant nausea, could not eat anything, her kidneys were failing, and she frequently drifted into a semi-conscious state.

As a last resort, the family decided to call in a doctor, known for his work along sound physiological principles.

The physician discontinued all medication except digitalis, ordered warm cleansing enemas and hot mustard foot baths, and for the first two days eliminated all food with the exception of two ounces of freshly squeezed grapefruit juice every two hours. Later, small meals of the foods mentioned in this book were permitted. Somewhat later, the digitalis was reduced to a bare minimum.

The change was dramatic. The kidneys began to function better almost immediately, and before long returned to normal, while the nausea and lack of appetite disap-

[3] "Medical Education To-Day," *JAMA,* March 20, 1944.

peared within a short time. The semi-conscious condition cleared up within two days and never returned.

The patient is now looking forward to her meals with keen interest. She sits up for hours at a time, has gained seven pounds in weight, is bright and cheerful, and is now wondering how soon she will be permitted to go outdoors.

"In view of the startling results obtained in this case within such a short time, who is there to say that the failure of the kidneys, as well as the other symptoms, were not induced by the medicines which were used in the treatment of the disease?" the physician remarked; and after reading Dr. Barr's report, who can say that the physician was wrong?

While most people are seldom aware of this, and while even doctors often fail to recognize it, it is nevertheless known that symptoms which are thought to be due to the disease are often actually caused by the medicines used in the treatment of the disease. This is why skilled doctors are often reluctant to prescribe drugs and why they often resort to "placebos" or "make-believe" drugs.

We would urge all physicians to read carefully Dr. Barr's thesis and pay particular attention to the sections dealing with the unforeseen complications that often arise from the use of drugs, as well as the increasing hazards when a multiplicity of drugs are used. Physicians must get away from the blind emphasis of relief of symptoms and must forever bear in mind that their first effort must be to determine the cause or causes of the disease, and then strive to remove or modify these causes and provide the care which will help in counteracting their effects.

CHAPTER XXII

A COMPLETELY INTEGRATED
PROGRAM ESSENTIAL

If the problem is really to be solved, all the factors which enter into the picture must receive serious attention.

We have seen from the tests conducted by New York University, Bellevue Medical Center, that American youngsters trail far behind European children in muscular fitness.[1]

The fact that nearly 50 percent of our young men were found unfit for military service is history. *U. S. News & World Report*[2] reported that out of 3.6 million American men under twenty-six years of age examined for military service between July 1950 to September 1953, 1.7 million, or nearly half, were rejected as unfit.

Further investigation will disclose that 9.3 percent of those rejected suffered from heart disease while another 5 percent suffered from high blood pressure.

Furthermore, we have seen from the report of Major General Dan C. Ogle that an examination of our boys who were killed in the Korean War, average age twenty-two, disclosed that 77.3 percent were suffering from diseased arteries.

It all adds up to one thing. With a poor beginning and a continuance of an unhealthful, although rich standard of living, no better results can be expected. No wonder investigations revealed that we have the "highest rate of heart disease than any other nation in the world."

[1] "What's Wrong with American Youths," *U. S. News & World Report*, March 19, 1954.
[2] *U. S. News & World Report*, October 4, 1955.

Blake Clark[3] in *Reader's Digest,* November, 1955, pointed out that Dr. Ancel Keys, in a study of coronary heart disease in many parts of the world, as related to the consumption of fat, found that the mortality in Italy "from degenerative heart disease in men is less than a third of ours," that in occupied Norway, where the fat supply was low as compared with Sweden which was unoccupied and whose fat supply was near normal standards "the coronary heart disease rate declined most," that the incidence of seriously diseased coronaries in Japan proved to be about one tenth of that in the U. S., and that checks in other countries proved that wherever the consumption of fat is high, a correspondingly high mortality from coronary heart disease exists, and that our mortality is highest because of the high consumption of fat in our diet.

While Dr. Keys' study stressed primarily the high level of fat consumption, we must not make the mistake of concentrating our attention on one factor only, disregarding all the other factors.

Problem Not Insoluble

From all the facts disclosed in this book, it should be clear that the problem is not insurmountable but that only when all the deleterious influences are recognized and removed, can it be brought under control.

We are happy to see Dr. Paul Dudley White, Dean of American heart specialists, pointing out that many of the factors, "about which we can do something, have received much too little study," mentioning "diet, tobacco, alcohol, exercise, stress and strain and local customs" among these factors. These factors must receive attention not when we are already advanced in years and when the foundation for the disease has already been laid, although they will be of help even then, but must become an integral part of our existence throughout life.

We cannot do better than quote Dr. Alexis Carrel who many years ago stated that "any true prolongation of life will require not only protection against disease but im-

---

[3] "Is This The No. 1 Villain in Heart Disease?"

provement of the quality of tissues and blood,"[4] and Dr. Edmund V. Cowdry of the Washington School of Medicine, who mentioned that what we need is not only medical help for aging persons, but also new measures which will help us prevent "a sizable number of ills and handicaps that otherwise will beset increasing millions of people."[5]

While we are interested in handling the diseases of the heart and blood vessels most efficiently, our major problem is to prevent their development, and this can easily be done through a reorganization of our daily habits of living.

We can do no better at this point than quote Dr. Shirley W. Wynne, who, as early as 1930, stated:

"The cause of arteriosclerosis is not at all clear. Some authorities claim that it results from the infectious diseases especially syphilis. Others blame tobacco. Others put it down to a diet containing too much protein and salt. . . . As it is frequently associated with chronic diseases of the heart and the kidneys, the well-regulated life which tends to prevent these diseases may likewise prevent this ailment."[6]

[4] "Carrel Urges Fund for Study of Aging," *New York Times,* Dec. 4, 1937.

[5] "Geriatrics Urged in Medical Schools," *New York Times,* August 28, 1953.

[6] *New York World,* May 25, 1930.

CHAPTER XXIII

A DECALOGUE OF HEALTH
FOR THE HEART SUFFERERS

By way of reminder, let us state that the body possesses vast recuperative powers which, if not abused, are of tremendous help even in the most difficult cases of heart disease. Here is a summary of the essentials which must be followed if we are to obtain maximum benefits in these cases:

1. Plenty of rest and sleep is imperative. In heart disease we are dealing with an overworked and badly injured heart, and its work must be reduced to a minimum, if it is to become strengthened and rebuilt.

2. The food of the sufferer from heart disease must be carefully controlled. The meals should be composed of simple, natural foods, the live foods, the foods which contain all the protective elements such as the vitamins, minerals and enzymes, in addition to all other essential nourishing elements required by the body. All processed and preserved foods, rich, concentrated, fat foods, seasoned foods, as well as all foods of a stimulating or irritating nature must be excluded.

Furthermore, the combinations must be of the simplest, since a mixture of too many foods at any one meal interferes with digestion, overtaxes the digestive organs, and places an added burden on the heart.

3. The quantity of food must be limited in these cases since this lessens the work of the heart and gives the body a chance to control weight, a factor which is of great importance in these cases. We are in complete agreement with the French proverb quoted by Bogomoletz that "to get fat is to get old."

4. Regular bowel functioning must be maintained. The many dietetic abuses extending over many years have made us a nation of constipated people. It is well to remember that the bowels act as an important organ of elimination, and when unable to function normally lead to the retention of waste products which produce putrefactive poisons and cause the formation of gas. This leads to pressure against the diaphragm which is directly underneath the heart, producing a strain on the heart as well as all other adjacent organs.

5. The use of drugs to induce sleep should be avoided since natural physiological methods can induce restful sleep without impairing our vital functions.

6. That a happy and cheerful disposition can do much to prolong life and keep us healthy is now well appreciated. Fear, insecurity, depression, impair the functions of our body, create much unhappiness and increase the burden on the heart. Cheerfulness, contentment, and a peaceful outlook on the other hand, promote good digestion and keep the body young and healthy.

7. Avoid all habits of a dissipating and health-destroying character. This includes the discontinuance of tobacco, liquor, an overindulgence in sweets, overeating, late hours, over-stimulation, excitement of various kinds, and excesses of all types.

8. Choose a sensible and relaxing hobby. It contributes to a serene and contented outlook and promotes a well-balanced life.

9. Don't overlook the benefits of exercise. While total or complete rest may be necessary during the acute stage of the disease or when the heart is at a very low ebb, properly regulated exercises or activities adjusted to the need and the ability of the patient can be of great help in strengthening and rebuilding the heart and circulation.

10. Finally, when in need of help, make sure that you avail yourself of the services of a doctor who is versed in the physiological approach and who possesses the knowledge, experience, and skill to help you through the difficult period successfully. In addition, he must also recognize the importance of teaching you to adhere to a sensible, well-balanced way of living as protection against the possibility of a reoccurrence of the condition.

CHAPTER XXIV

A SAMPLE PROGRAM

The following is a reproduction of a program sent to a patient suffering from a chronic heart condition. While this program cannot be followed indiscriminately, since the measures employed in each case must be carefully evaluated, it nevertheless serves as an illustration of what a basic approach in such cases should be.

1. *Eat Sparingly*

   Small meals do not overtax the digestion and save the heart from overwork.

2. *Eat Simple Meals*

   Avoid fancy desserts and sauces, all rich foods, and do not use too many dishes at any one meal.

   Omit completely all fat foods, all spices and condiments, all sweets, all white flour and white sugar products, coffee and tea.

   Eliminate fried foods and don't use chilled foods.

3. *Do not take liquids or liquid foods with your meals.*

4. *Make sure to take a complete rest after each meal.*

5. *See that you get plenty of rest and sleep.*

   A nap after the noon meal is of great help.

6. *Relax Completely*

   Avoid tension and emotional upsets.

   Calmness, poise, and emotional control are essential to the rebuilding of health.

7. *Bowels must be kept functioning regularly.*

   When necessary, small enemas should be taken.

8. *Warm baths before retiring induce relaxation and in most cases help bring on restful sleep.*

   (Where for any reason the full bath cannot be used, the hot mustard foot bath, if permissible in the case, can be of great help.)

9. *Do Everything Slowly and Be of Good Cheer.*
   Eat slowly, talk slowly, and do everything slowly.
   Never do anything to excess.
10. *Always keep your feet warm and your head emotionally cool.*

A SEVEN DAY MENU

We have seen that the diet for the sufferer from heart and blood vessel diseases varies in accordance with the condition and the needs of the case. At times the diet has to be greatly restricted, while at other times a more liberal food intake is permissible. This is the reason we emphasize that the diet, as well as all other care, be subject to the supervision of the doctor who has an understanding of the patient's requirements and who is conversant with the latest nutritional concepts as well as the hygienic principles of healing.

In view of this, it should be apparent that the seven day menu which we are presenting on these pages is not meant for those who require special care but is offered merely as an illustration to indicate what the diet should be where no special supervision is necessary.

SUNDAY

Breakfast:

> Grated or shredded raw apple (slightly heated).
> *Buckwheat groats.
> 4-6 ounces of raw skimmed milk.
> 4-5 medium sized stewed prunes.

Lunch:

> Waldorf Salad of diced apple, pear, ripe pineapple, pascal celery. Add a few natural raisins and strawberries in season. Serve on lettuce leaves with 3-4 ounces of cottage cheese.
> Stewed fresh peaches or soaked unsulphured dry peaches.

Dinner:

> Salad of grated carrots, chopped lettuce, grated or shredded cucumber, a sprig of watercress.

Bowl of natural brown rice with steamed polebeans or stringbeans.
Compote of fresh stewed fruits.

MONDAY

Breakfast:

½ grapefruit.
Heated apples and blueberries.
Baked banana.
4-6 ounces of skimmed milk, clabbered or soured milk or yoghurt (sipped slowly or eaten with a spoon).

Lunch:

Salad of lettuce, tomatoes and shredded cucumber.
Lentils steamed or baked with celery and carrots (with leek or onion for flavoring), and steamed stringbeans.
Stewed fresh or soaked dry unsulphured apricots.

Dinner:

Salad of finely grated cabbage, grated beets, diced pascal celery, with the addition of a few raisins.
Vegetable stew of carrots, parsnips, squash and stringbeans.
Baked potato.
Stewed pears.

TUESDAY

Breakfast:

Sliced peaches and blueberries, heated.
Shredded wheat (eaten with stewed fruit).
4-6 ounces of raw skimmed milk, clabbered or soured milk or yoghurt.

Lunch:

Salad of grated carrots, escarole, diced green pepper, grated parsnips, a sprig of watercress.
Wild rice with sauce of stewed celery, green pepper and onion, steamed green peas and carrots.
Baked apple filled with raisins.

Dinner:

Salad of lettuce, grated beets, endive, sliced cucumber.

Baked potato, steamed eggplant (with onion and celery for flavoring).
Compote of fresh stewed fruits.

WEDNESDAY

Breakfast:
Raw apple and raspberries, heated.
Natural brown rice with diced apple and natural raisins.
4-6 ounces of raw skimmed milk, clabbered or soured milk or yoghurt.

Lunch:
Fruit salad of diced honeydew, cantaloupe balls, diced ripe pineapple, balls of watermelon. Add a sprinkling of raisins. Served on a bed of lettuce leaves with 3-4 ounces of farmer cheese or ricotta cheese.
Grated raw apple and raisins.

Dinner:
Salad of grated white turnips, grated half-cooked beets, grated raw carrots, served in balls on lettuce leaves.
Baked yams, steamed okra (steamed with onion and tomato for flavoring), green peas and carrots.
Baked pear.

THURSDAY

Breakfast:
Stewed blueberries and apple.
Baked banana.
4-6 ounces of raw skimmed milk, clabbered or soured milk or yoghurt.

Lunch:
Lettuce, tomato, and chicory salad.
Steamed lentils (onions and celery for added flavor), steamed kale, baked butternut squash.
Stewed apricots or any other stewed fresh or soaked dry unsulphured fruit.

Dinner:
Salad of lettuce, grated beets, escarole, strips of cucumber.

Baked potato, steamed kale, steamed or baked pumpkin.
Any stewed fruit for dessert.

FRIDAY

Breakfast:
Fruit salad of apples, bananas, pears and blueberries.
4-6 ounces of raw skimmed milk or clabbered or soured milk or yoghurt.

Lunch:
Spring salad of finely diced cucumbers, diced radishes (used sparingly primarily to add color), diced green pepper, finely diced scallions, served on lettuce leaves with 3-4 ounces of farmer cheese or cottage cheese.
Steamed beets and steamed broccoli.
½ grapefruit.

Dinner:
Salad of finely grated cabbage, grated carrots, grated beets, strips of green pepper.
Young tender corn on cob, prepared as per instructions, steamed eggplant (steamed with celery and onion), steamed stringbeans.
Baked apple.

SATURDAY

Breakfast:
Blueberries and sliced peaches, heated.
*Buckwheat groats.
4-6 ounces of raw skimmed milk.
4-5 medium sized stewed prunes.

Lunch:
Tomatoes stuffed with cottage cheese, garnished with watercress and parsley, served on lettuce leaves, with strips of carrots and cucumber on the side.
Steamed beets, baked acorn squash.
Compote of fresh stewed fruits.

Dinner:
Salad of grated raw cauliflower, finely diced green pepper, diced celery and apple.

Stew of white potato, yams, stewed prunes and raisins, steamed stringbeans.
Stewed pears.

You will note that we endeavor to keep the meals as simple as possible and that we do not recommend too great a variety of foods at one time. Too many foods eaten together overtax the digestion and should, therefore, be avoided.

A raw vegetable salad should be used at least once daily, unless contra-indicated because of digestive difficulties. We have pointed out before that the unheated or uncooked foods provide much valuable nourishment and where conditions permit, these foods should make up a great part of the menu.

As a rule, we prefer that no meat or fish be included in the diet. However, those who feel that they cannot do without these foods may use small portions of chicken, lambchops, or lean fish, or any lean meat, in place of cheese or lentils. When meat or fish is included in the diet, it should be used at most three times a week.

Substitutions of vegetables or fruits in season for those not available or difficult to obtain will help vary the meals and make them more pleasurable.

The following steamed or baked vegetables may be substituted for one another: parsnips, carrots, beets, turnips, celery, leek, kale, okra, beet greens, zucchini, butternut squash, acorn squash, pumpkin, green peas, stringbeans, asparagus, artichokes, swisschard, broccoli.

No sugar should be added to the fruit. No salt or butter should be used. Steamed vegetables may be flavored by the addition of dill, tomato, onion, leek, garlic, celery, sage, anise, sweet basil, rosemary, caraway seeds. The use of these natural flavorings can be developed into quite an art. Use them sparingly, merely to enhance the natural flavors of the food, not to drown them out.

A dressing of lemon and honey may be added to the fruit and vegetable salads for flavoring purposes. A dressing of tomato juice, cottage cheese, lemon juice and honey, with or without the addition of garlic, will enhance the flavor of the raw vegetable salad. Sweet paprika may also be used for garnishing purposes on either the raw or steamed vegetables.

If still hungry, you may use a yam or baked banana with the stewed fruit for dessert.

Milk, clabbered or soured milk or yoghurt should be sipped slowly or taken with a spoon. Remove cream from clabbered milk.

Acidophilus milk is an excellent milk food and could be used in place of the above.

Use only raw skimmed milk whenever possible.

*How to Prepare Buckwheat Groats

Use 2½ parts of water to one part of groats. Bring water to a boil. Add groats. Cover pot and turn off the flame. A few raisins may be added. Let stand for twenty to twenty-five minutes until the water is soaked up. It is then ready to serve. Of the three types of groats available in the market, the coarse or medium groats are to be preferred.

In some cases, a small amount of honey may be added to the groats when serving, to enhance the flavor. The groats may be eaten with stewed fruit, or raw skimmed milk may be added.

Corn on the cob should be boiled not longer than one to two minutes. Keep pot covered. Turn off flame and keep in boiling water for another five minutes before serving.

Grapefruit and other citrus fruits should be used only when fully ripe to avoid the harsh irritating acids they contain during the early part of the citrus fruit season. These fruits are frequently subjected to gassing and the addition of color to make them appear ripe.

Noon and evening meals may be interchanged.

The diet outlined above is subject to many variations. A more ideal diet would be one in which the breakfast would be composed exclusively of raw fresh fruit or would be omitted altogether, limiting the menu to two meals a day.

An even more restricted diet, omitting the first two meals, using grapefruit only about every two or three hours, finishing the day with the regular evening meal, if followed for a day or two at a time, can be of great help in many cases. A variation of this program, using any kind of fresh fruit every two or three hours and ending the day with the regular evening meal, is also of great help in many cases.

Remember that complete abstinence from food for a day or two or even a longer period often saves human life.

The Following Rules Must Be Carefully Observed:

1. Eat slowly.
2. Eat only when hungry.
3. Do not overeat (small meals).
4. Do not eat between meals.
5. Do not eat when disturbed or emotionally upset.

Other Points of Importance

No smoking, no liquor, no carbonated drinks!

Small servings of apple juice, unsweetened grape juice, or any freshly squeezed unsweetened fruit juice may be taken between meals if desired and if conditions allow it.

A sound health-building program must be followed consistently if good results are to be attained. However, it is imperative that the program outlined in the individual case conform to the needs of the case. This is why we stress the need of careful supervision.

A menu presented in print, even at its best, is but a poor substitute for a diet worked out to suit the temperament, the habits and the needs of the individual case. Guidance, furthermore, helps to do a more thorough job and removes some of the uncertainties as well as the difficulties which may present themselves to one who is not acquainted with this way of living.

However, those who are not in position to avail themselves of personal care will, provided they have no special problem requiring individual attention, benefit tremendously by changing from the conventional diet to the menu presented above.

It is evident that the meals outlined in the above menu are quite different from those served in the average home. Some may wonder how satisfying they are, as well as how difficult they are to prepare. In reply to this, we wish to point out that much less time is required for the preparation of these meals, while so far as taste is concerned, most people find them extremely satisfying and pleasurable. Just give it a good try and see how enjoyable these meals can be. Furthermore, they will pay off immeasurably in improved health!

CHAPTER XXV

CONCLUSION

Fifty Years Ahead of Our Time

Doctors as well as the public at large are finally awakening to the realization that what we eat and how we live determines to a great extent whether we are rapidly building up towards a heart attack, a stroke or some of the conditions which ultimately lead to one of these life-taking tragedies, or whether if we keep ourselves well and strong and we will live to a healthy, ripe old age.

Dr. William D. Kannel, a distinguished scientist, director of one of the National Heart Institute teams, engaged in the study of how these life-destroying ills can be prevented, aptly stated: "Heart attacks are not entirely natural; they are to a large extent man created, and if the knowledge we have now were properly applied, we could halve the number of deaths from coronary attacks. In short we could probably save 200,000 lives a year."[1]

Here in this book we have given you the knowledge, the wisdom how you can apply yourself, how you can plan your way of living, so that you can protect yourself against these life-threatening ills and build a long and healthy life. The rest is up to you. If you are wise, you will adopt this way of living and make it a life-time proposition so that you may add years to your life and life to your years.

[1] *Reader's Digest*, April 1969.